Food Allergies

Food Allergies

- ## How to Tell if You Have Them
- ## What to Do About Them if You Do

Neil S. Orenstein, Ph.D., and
Sarah L. Bingham, M.S.

A Perigee Book

This book deals with the important relationship between food and allergy. It is intended to serve as a general information guide and as a reference source. Responsibility for any adverse effects or unforeseen consequences resulting from the use of any information contained herein is expressly disclaimed, and rests solely with the reader.

Perigee Books
are published by
The Putnam Publishing Group
200 Madison Avenue
New York, NY 10016

"Possible Common Symptoms of Allergy" chart reprinted, modified, from *Allergies and the Hyperactive Child,* copyright © 1979 by Doris J. Rapp, by permission of Simon & Schuster, Inc.

Library of Congress Cataloging-in-Publication Data

Orenstein, Neil S.
  Food allergies.

  "A Perigee book."
  Bibliography: p.
  1. Food allergy—Diet therapy. I. Bingham, Sarah L.
II. Title.
RC596.074 1987   616.97'5   87-10926
ISBN 0-399-51383-3

Printed in the United States of America

1 2 3 4 5 6 7 8 9 10

TO WILLIAM G. CROOK, M.D.
whose dedication and teachings have inspired
laymen and nutrition professionals
throughout the world.

ACKNOWLEDGMENTS

Many thanks:
to the wonderful culinary artists who have made The Culinary Arts Center possible: Mary Theresa Valleri, Julia Herman, Bianca Fiore, Robin Wade, Kathie Maye, Joanne O'Neil, Indra Milowe, and Pamela Usenza;

to Carol Polizzi for sharing the allergy-free recipes that were a hit with her son;

to William for trying out some very unusual recipes;

to Noreen Blair for putting up with a difficult typing project;

to Judy Linden, our editor at Putnam's, for her support and excellent suggestions;

to Theresa DiGeronimo for her untiring assistance, organizational skills, and expertise in helping us with this book.

Contents

Contents

Our drug-culture society should begin to appreciate that not all human misery can be alleviated by "taking something." Sometimes it is better to remove the "something" that initiates the suffering.

Basics of Food Allergy, 1984
James C. Breneman, M.D.

1 · Food Allergies

Discovering a hidden food allergy is like opening a door to find a future filled with good health and vitality on the other side. The food allergy detection program that we will outline in this book is your key to unlocking that door. We call it the Simplification Diet Program—and it works!

Both of us began our work with food allergies as skeptics. In the early 1970s, Neil worked in the traditional medical research settings of the Harvard School of Public Health, Massachusetts General Hospital, Beth Israel Hospital in Boston, and Harvard Medical School. At the time, it seemed absurd to him that any major medical health problem could be caused by an adverse reaction to food. Then in 1980 he joined a study group along with twenty nutritionally oriented medical doctors. In addition, Neil slowly began to see that the writings of nutritional practitioners such as Sidney Baker, M.D., William Crook, M.D., and Jonathan Wright, M.D., were correct in claiming that not only were food allergies widespread, but that the majority of their patients had one or more food allergies, and that many suffered major medical problems because of them.

After listening to the members of the study group regularly praise simplification diets, and after watching scores of people find good health for the first time in their lives through these diets, Neil became a believer. Now, in his own practice as a nutritional biochemist, Neil finds that over half of his clients have one or more food allergies. He uses the simplification concept with these clients through his Simplification Diet Program, finding this method to be his most powerful and successful tool for bringing these people to good health.

Sarah, on the other hand, came into the field of nutrition after a trip around the world left her with dysentery, ulcers, and fatigue. When a doctor prescribed Valium as the only remedy for her pain, Sarah set out to find a better way to good health. After trying a nutritional approach to her problems, she saw for herself the profound healing effect that a change in diet can bring. Now, with nine years' experience as a nutrition consultant, Sarah has learned that each of us has a unique response to the foods we eat. She has seen the truth in the old saying, "One man's meat is another man's poison."

As founder of the Culinary Arts Center in Lenox, Massachusetts, Sarah has taught hundreds of people how to discover the foods that cause negative reactions in their bodies, and how to cook healthy, allergen-free foods. Ninety percent of her clients have found relief from their symptoms with this Simplification Diet Program—and so can you.

The two of us have seen how difficult it can be for new ideas to be accepted by the medical establishment. This actually makes sense: it is right for medicine to move ahead cautiously and deliberately, accepting new ideas only as their validity is confirmed.

We are very pleased that, parallel to our own experiences, medical research has now proved the importance of considering food allergies in the diagnosis of ailments, and medical publications have detailed the role food allergies play in health problems. Because of this, many more professionals involved in traditional medical practices are now prescribing simplification-type diets to their patients.

Others, however, still prescribe drugs, recommend surgery, or declare a "no-cure" situation when, in fact, many of their patients could be quickly "cured" of their symptoms through a simplification diet. This professional reluctance lies, in part, in the controversy over the term "food allergy." Many doctors, and even allergists, claim that "food allergy" is properly used when describing symptoms caused only by the specific type of immunological reactions in which immunoglobulin E (IgE) is involved. This kind of food reaction occurs in a mere two percent of the population. Because most adverse reactions to food do not involve this IgE component and therefore do not fit into the "correct" technical definition, a more fitting term for their occurrence is "food sensitivity." However, for the purposes of this book, and because for the general public "allergy" is a significant and recognizable term, we have decided to use the term "food allergy" to describe *all* adverse reactions to food, IgE-mediated or not.

These kinds of food allergies know no bounds. They strike regardless of age, nationality, occupation, or family history. An important factor in determining whether or not you have food allergies is often the condition of your digestive system. So that you can better understand how this happens we'll explain the digestive process as having three simplified components: the first is chewing and predigestion by enzymes in our mouths; the second is digestion by acid in our stomachs; and the third is digestion by enzymes in our intestines. Each of these three (mouth, stomach, and intestine) needs to function well for food to be completely digested and absorbed in a healthy manner, and to prevent food allergies.

Chewing is obviously important. There is much talk about chewing well, eating slowly, and giving the digestive process a head start. In addition to beginning the food breakdown process, the act of chewing, combined with the senses of taste and smell, stimulates our other digestive organs and primes them for action.

The next step of digestion, acidification of foods in the stomach, plays two very important roles. First, it "predigests" food, particularly protein; second, it stimulates our pancreas to begin the next phase of digestion, the enzymatic process in our intestines. In response to acid made by our stomach, our pancreas secretes into the upper portion of our intestine a whole host of enzymes, which complete the digestion process. We usually think that most problems in this portion of our digestive tract are caused by too much stomach acid. But, in fact, undersecretion of stomach acid is probably more problematic than oversecretion or excess stomach acidity. Low stomach acid both prevents the predigestion of foods in the stomach (particularly protein) and reduces pancreatic stimulation, thus also inhibiting the enzymatic or third stage of digestion in the intestines.

How does all this relate to food allergies? The answer is quite simple. Your immune system does not recognize your own body, and immunologists call this concept nonrecognition of self. Foreign substances are recognized as "nonself" and are attacked by your immune system. This is how the defensive immune system is able to protect us from the invasion of harmful bacteria and viruses: it recognizes these invaders as "nonself," mounts an attack, and destroys the bacteria.

The food we eat is basically "nonself." Vegetables and animal-derived foods have very little in common chemically with our own bodies. If our immune system were to take a close look at these substances, they would certainly be considered "nonself," and our immune system would actually attack the foods we eat. The way nature gets around this problem is to ensure that the digestive process reduces the foods we eat to sufficiently small molecules so that these food components, after digestion, are not seen as foreign and no immune attack is mounted. But if we don't chew well in the first stage of the digestive process, and then don't make enough stomach acid to predigest our food, thus, in turn, not stimulating pancreatic enzyme activity in our intestines to further digest our food, we end up with large molecules of food in our intestine. These large molecules then pass through the intestinal wall and are circulated in our bloodstream, incompletely digested and nonetheless absorbed. This then triggers an immune attack because our immune system thinks the food is an invading pathogen. This confusion and overreaction on the part of the immune system results in the symptoms of food allergies.

The way we experience these symptoms is largely determined by our individual genetic makeup. An allergy to wheat may be expressed in one person as a headache, in another as diarrhea, in another as aching joints, in yet another as asthma or breathing difficulties, and so on. Our allergic response is also of different types. The first is the immediate onset type, in which symptoms occur within seconds to minutes of ingesting a food. Because the symptoms occur immediately and in an explosive manner, a relationship between the food and the reaction is unquestionable. You usually don't need diets or tests to confirm this kind of food allergy. The second type of response is that of delayed onset, in which symptoms occur several hours to several days after ingestion of food. With this type of delayed reaction, tests for the IgE component are usually negative. Thus, even after a medical consultation and laboratory testing, you might not see a connection between your symptoms and a food allergy.

Our goal in writing this book is to prevent this from happening to you. The Simplification Diet Program will give you the information you need to determine once and for all (regardless of your previous medical diagnosis and treatments) if you suffer from a food allergy. It will help you identify the particular food or foods that are causing your distress, and it will offer diet suggestions and recipes that will allow you to be vigorous, full of energy, and free from the effects of food allergies.

2 · An Overview of the Simplification Diet Program

When you picked up this book, you made an important decision to gain control of your own health and well-being. Maybe you've decided to investigate food allergies because you're tired of taking aspirin for your chronic headaches. Or perhaps you no longer believe that diarrhea, constipation, excessive gas, or bloating are an unavoidable part of your life. Does your fatigue, skin problems, or breathing difficulties now force you to miss out on some of life's good times? Whatever your personal reason, we're delighted that, like the hundreds of other people we have worked with in our private practices, you are ready to explore food allergies as the possible cause of your symptoms.

THE SIMPLIFICATION DIET PROGRAM IS DIFFERENT FROM OTHER PROGRAMS

The process involved in the Simplification Diet Program is not a new one. For many years the medical community has recognized food allergies as the cause of innumerable physical and psychological ailments. Programs that have grown out of this knowledge, however, are often complicated and difficult to follow and some-times inaccurate. Some rely on laboratory tests to identify food allergies, but most of these tests have not yet been perfected. It is very common for these allergy tests to give false results. Tests such as RAST and cytotoxic testing (blood tests), skin testing, sublingual (beneath the tongue) testing, and modifications of these techniques can err in two ways: they may report that you are allergic to a food to which, in fact, you are not; or they may give a false reading and label as "safe" a food to which you are actually allergic. Although a new test presently being developed may improve the rate of accuracy, most tests only measure a portion of the whole chain of events involved in an allergic reaction. It is possible that the test used on you does not measure the part of your biochemistry and immune system that is reacting. Eggs, for example, can cause more than one type of allergic reaction, one of which may not be picked up by laboratory tests. You may have a standard type (IgE) of immunological reaction to the protein in the egg and get the ap-propriate positive result from the lab test. But in some people egg protein is also capable of bypassing this traditional immune-mediated reaction although it still causes allergic symptoms. In this case you would get a negative lab result even though you are having a genuine allergic reaction. Our program uses your entire body as the testing ground with no possibility of missing an allergic reaction. The Simplification Diet Program is foolproof.

Other programs treat food allergies with drug therapy. We be-lieve, however, that drugs only serve to dull the symptoms, and they hinder attempts to find the underlying cause of your problem. The drugs used to treat allergies (such as antihistamines, bron-chodilators, corticosteroids, and decongestants) often have side ef-fects: drowsiness, anxiety, frequent and painful urination, nausea, vomiting, dry mouth, loss of appetite, abdominal discomfort and cramps, constipation or diarrhea, or headaches. Not only are these side effects difficult to bear, but they make it difficult to separate the body's food allergy reaction from its drug reaction. Both com-monly problematic foods and over-the-counter drugs are cleared from the body's system in the Simplification Diet Program.

Another popular method of treating food allergies is with a rotation diet. This involves a complex routine of rotating and often color-coding the foods in your cabinets and refrigerator. By continually clearing your system of commonly problematic foods, allergy symptoms may sometimes be relieved, but this approach does not necessarily pinpoint the particular food that is causing your adverse reaction, as you could be eating two foods you are reactive to on the same day. But on the Simplification Diet Program, you will be able to identify the food, or foods, that you are allergic to one by one and you can learn how to use this knowledge to find a new health.

You may have already found that some allergy detection programs are very expensive and lengthy. The program presented in this book is a self-help approach that is easy to use, quick to show results in seven days, and very inexpensive. By the seventh day, most people who have allergies can see clear evidence of it.

THE STRENGTHS OF THIS PROGRAM

Unlike some of the methods we've just described, the Simplification Diet Program is totally accurate because you will measure the end results of a whole series of reactions. The chain of events includes eating the food, absorbing the digested food, and distributing the digested food via the bloodstream to all the tissues and organs of the body, including the immune system. If something goes wrong along the way and triggers an allergic reaction you'll know it. There are no false results when you test the foods directly on your own body.

The Simplification Diet Program is a general program that works despite the vast differences in each individual's allergic reactions:

- The program will work for you if your allergy causes symptoms that are merely annoying, such as a headache or fatigue, as well as for more severe reactions.
- It will work if your reaction to a problem food is immediate; it will also work if the food takes several hours or even days to trigger an attack.
- The program will work for you if you react adversely after eating just a tiny morsel, as well as if you react only after eating larger quantities.

- It will work whether you were born with your immunological sensitivity to a particular food or you've developed your allergy recently.
- The program also works if your allergies are additive, that is, if the problem food only causes an adverse reaction when it is taken in combination with something else that is also stressing your immune system. For instance, your allergy is additive if you get hives only when you eat a particular food while the pollen count is high, or you are emotionally upset, or you're fighting off the flu. This program will help you too.

FOOD ALLERGIES ARE MORE COMMON THAN YOU THINK

The food allergy problem is quite widespread and steadily growing. William T. Kniker, M.D., head of clinical immunology at the University of Texas Health Science Center, says that countless millions of Americans suffer from undiagnosed food allergies. In fact, many medical authorities are convinced that the problem has increased substantially over the past fifty years. One possible reason for this is the lack of variety in a steady diet of processed foods. Even though these foods look different, taste different, and have different textures and flavors, they almost always contain one or more of the most commonly allergenic ingredients: corn (syrup), egg (white), milk solids, yeast, and wheat or soy derivatives. Our ancestors ate a much more varied diet. They hadn't as efficient a system for food storage as refrigeration, and processed foods were unknown. They ate a seasonal diet made up of foods grown or hunted locally. This is no longer true. Now medical research reports a link between food allergies and increased consumption of processed foods.

In addition, processed foods commonly contain artificial colorings such as tartrazine dye (yellow dye no. 5), as well as artificial preservatives such as benzoic acid, BHA, and BHT. Each of these may also cause food allergies. One mother brought her son, Mark, to me because he was having great difficulty in school. He suffered from restlessness, a short attention span, and behavioral problems.

His doctor had suggested the use of behavior-modification drugs, but his mother hoped there was another way to solve her son's problems. With the Simplification Diet Program we found Mark was allergic to foods containing preservatives and artificial colorings. Without these foods in his diet, Mark's behavioral problems disappeared and he went on to become a good student. That sounds like a happy ending, but remember that fifty years ago Mark would not have suffered from behavioral problems because the foods causing his problem didn't even exist.

Another possible reason for a historical increase in food allergies is that our immune systems have become weaker over the last seventy-five years. If your immune system is balanced, you will not have any allergies or other health-related immune problems. But if your immune system is weakened so that it is overactive and reacts too frequently, problems will arise. Mild forms of overreaction are seasonal allergies, such as hay fever. As the weakened immune system continues overreacting, our discomfort increases and we may react to more and more allergens, including foods. One of the most important things we can do to keep our immune system balanced is to have adequate nutrients in our diet.

Dr. R. K. Chandra, a food allergy specialist formerly of the Massachusetts Institute of Technology, has done extensive research to show that the nutrients zinc and vitamin A are essential for strong immune systems. Other medical researchers have demonstrated that the B complex vitamins; vitamin C; vitamin E; the minerals, iron, copper, magnesium, iodine, and selenium; as well as high quality dietary protein are very important for strong immune systems. Yet a study documenting the changing trends in food consumption in the United States reports that the average person is consuming smaller amounts of food containing these nutrients, and larger amounts of nonnutritive high-sugar, high-fat food than our grandparents did seventy-five years ago.

Some results of the report from the United States Department of Agriculture are printed below. Six problem nutrients are listed to illustrate this point. Although the study found many other nutrients which are deficient in our diets, this small group of six makes it apparent that the typical American diet is not capable of consistently maintaining a strong immune system.

NUTRIENT DEFICIENCY IN THE UNITED STATES

Nutrient	Percent of Diets Providing Less Than 100% of the RDA
Calcium	68
Iron	57
Magnesium	75
Vitamin A	50
Vitamin B$_6$	80
Vitamin C	41

Is it any mystery that so many of us have food allergies when, as a population, we are no longer consuming the nutrients that are necessary to build and to maintain strong immune systems?

THE SYMPTOMS OF FOOD ALLERGIES

Whatever may be the exact reasons for their occurrence, food allergies are a medical reality that cause a wide range of symptoms. The problems most often associated with food allergies are:

- fatigue
- chronic crying and colic in children
- headache (include migraine)
- aches and pains in arms and legs
- anxiety
- behavioral problems in children
- vaginal discharge
- fluid retention
- chronic running and/or stuffed nose
- joint aches and pains
- skin problems including eczema, hives, rash, and dry and flaky skin
- diarrhea and/or constipation; digestive problems including excessive gas, bloating and abdominal pain
- breathing difficulties ranging from shortness of breath to severe asthma, including "exercise-induced asthma" (breathing difficulty during exercise), an extremely common problem
- seizures.

Scientific Evidence

The store of scientific and medical research supporting the connection between these symptoms and food allergies is growing daily. Studies such as the 1983 report on migraine headaches by Dr. Egger and his associates in London consistently support the view that there is a link between the foods we eat and physical ailments.

Dr. Egger studied eighty-eight children who suffered from frequent severe migraine headaches. The children were put on a simplification-type diet and their symptoms were monitored. Amazingly, 93 percent of these children suffered no migraines so long as they avoided the foods to which they were allergic.

Some of the foods that provoked the children's headaches are listed below. In certain cases, more than one food caused the headaches.

MIGRAINE-PRODUCING FOODS IN DR. EGGER'S STUDY

Food	Percent of Children Affected
Cow's milk	31
Egg	27
Chocolate	25
Orange	24
Wheat	24
Benzoic acid	16
Cheese	15
Tomato	15
Tartrazine (yellow dye no. 5)	14
Rye	14
Fish	10
Beef	10
Pork	9
Corn	9

In addition to showing that migraines could be the result of eating foods to which an individual is sensitive, the study demonstrated something that may be even more important. The simplification diet that reduced these headaches also reduced abdominal pain in 87 percent of the children, as well as aches in the limbs by 83 percent, chronic runny nose by 56 percent, vaginal discharge by 91 percent, asthma by 57 percent, eczema by 50 percent, and seizures by 86 percent. These improvements were accomplished with the relatively simple procedure of removing specific foods from the children's diets.

This same research group, headed by Dr. Egger, published another report in 1985 as a follow-up to their first study. In this project they tested seventy-six children who displayed hyperactivity, a serious behavioral disorder that handicaps children so that they have difficulty both studying effectively in school and interacting with others. The research found that the behavioral problems of 79 percent of the studied children improved substantially when foods to which they were sensitive were removed from their diets. And again, concurrent symptoms—headaches, abdominal pain, chronic runny nose, aches in limbs, and skin problems—were also greatly reduced while the children were on this diet.

Based on the results of studies like Dr. Egger's, many people have begun looking seriously at food allergies as a possible explanation for chronic and "untreatable" symptoms. Another study conducted by Dr. V. Alun Jones and her colleagues at the University of Cambridge in 1982 found that food allergies also play a major role in irritable bowel syndrome, the most common complaint of adult patients referred to physicians specializing in gastroenterology. The cause of irritable bowel syndrome is generally believed to be unknown but it usually results in abdominal pain accompanied by diarrhea, or constipation, and/or gas. The authors found that specific foods provoked symptoms of irritable bowel syndrome in fourteen of twenty-one patients studied. In our own experience, we have found the Simplification Diet Program to be the end of a long search for many people who couldn't find the cause or the cure for their digestive distress.

In 1985 Dr. D. J. Atherton reported research findings in the *Journal of the Royal Society of Medicine* that complemented the study published in the *Medical Journal of Australia* that same year by doctors A. S. Kemp and G. Schembri. These reports noted remarkable improvement in the control of hives and eczema through simplification diets. In our experience we too have found that the symptoms associated with skin disease can be greatly reduced or even eliminated through the Simplification Diet Program.

After using our program, one mother wrote us: "At the age of three, my oldest son, Dylan, still had the dry patchy skin he had since birth. It was diagnosed as eczema. The eczema on his worst spots, wrists, hands, feet, knees, and the back of his legs, got so out of control it spread to all parts of his arms, legs, face, and even his penis. He would scratch all night long. Dylan never slept for more than one hour at a time. I would find blood underneath his fingernails and on the sheets. He would walk around with his wrists so dry he would bleed. His face was constantly swollen and puffy. He looked diseased all over his body. Our physicians were just at the point of starting Dylan on oral steroids to control his eczema when I decided to try the Simplification Diet Program. It worked! In Dylan's case, the eczema was caused by eggs, oats, chocolate, butter, artificial colorings (especially the yellow ones which we also found in shampoo and toothpaste), milk, and cottage cheese. Now, at age three and a half, Dylan's skin and body finally look normal. He sleeps all night and is a much happier child. He has learned to say no to a food he knows will make him scratch—even when it's a piece of chocolate cake offered at a birthday party!"

Another recent study by Dr. L. G. Darlington, involving 53 arthritis patients from Surrey, England, emphasized the effects of simplification diets on rheumatoid arthritis. During the time that problem foods were eliminated from their diets, there was objective, statistically significant improvement in arthritis symptoms. Pain, duration of morning stiffness, and the number of painful joints decreased, and grip strength increased.

Actor James Coburn also sought treatment for a food allergy after he completed a movie in Mexico. His arthritis was so bad during the filming that he could hardly move; they had to lift him on and off horses with a crane. Coburn's condition was dramatically improved by eliminating problem foods from his diet. He remarked during a December 1981 appearance on the "Merv Griffin Show" that the diet had saved his life. Reports like these, and our own findings, have brought hope to thousands of people suffering the chronic pain of arthritis.

Another problem that has responded well to simplification diets is fluid retention. This common sign of food allergies offers a very valuable self-assessment tool. If you find that you can gain or lose two pounds or more overnight, it is obvious that this weight fluctuation is not due to an increase or decrease in body fat. One of our clients was an overweight woman who lost eight pounds in the first week on the Simplification Diet. To have lost that weight in body fat, she would have had to have reduced her caloric intake or burned calories through exercise in excess of 28,000 calories, which is clearly impossible. This, combined with the fact that she urinated much more than usual during the week of the Simplification Diet, is a clear indication that most of those eight pounds were fluid. Because a drastic weight loss without a change in caloric intake almost always indicates a food allergy, you will be asked to keep careful track of your weight during the Simplification Diet Program.

Another symptom that requires a bit of self-analysis is anxiety. All people feel some degree of anxiety in their daily lives. This does not mean that everyone has a food allergy. You can begin to suspect a chemical reaction to foods, however, if your anxiety manifests itself in inappropriate fits of anger, or in hair-trigger emotional outbursts. Because we are not used to relating the things we do to the foods we eat, the food diary that is recommended in chapter three will be a great help in discerning whether or not your anxiety is caused by allergy.

As all adults feel anxiety at some point, so do all babies cry. But there is a point when the crying becomes excessive and thus an indication that something is wrong beyond hunger, cold, dirty diapers, or boredom. That something is very often "colic," the broad definition of which is inconsolable crying for which no physical cause can be found. This crying lasts for more than three hours a day, occurs at least three days a week, and continues for at least three weeks.

The exact cause of colic is debatable, but we have seen many times that the cure is found in the elimination of certain foods. A change of formula is sometimes all that is needed to calm the intestinal distress that most often accompanies a colic attack. Often a change from cow's milk to soy milk will do the trick. A recent study has found that even mother's milk can sometimes cause a reaction: some infants may actually be allergic to their own mother's milk if she is drinking cow's milk. (The details of this study are given in chapter seven.) We believe that food allergies should be considered a cause for any child's excessive crying and/or colic symptoms.

One mother of a crying baby discovered that her son was suffering from food allergies. His ailment, however, wasn't colic, but rather asthma. Little Devin was hospitalized after his first asthma attack when he was two weeks old. In the following eighteen months, he was hospitalized seven times more. Each time, he was put in an oxygen tent with an intravenous drip of steroids and aminophylline. He received respiratory treatments every four hours around the clock, and often the doctors would order tubes inserted in his nose to suction out the phlegm. Between hospitalizations, Devin would frequently have to be rushed to the emergency room to be treated with shots of adrenaline for an asthma attack.

At home, Devin always appeared pale; he coughed constantly and was irritable and panicky. His breathing was very wheezy and labored; you could hear him breathe from two rooms away.

Devin was eventually put on a Pulmo-aide machine at home with three prescription drugs to be inhaled every four hours. His mother was also told to wash the floors, walls, and crib in his room twice a day. The carpets, curtains, stuffed animals, and overstuffed furniture was removed from the house to cut down on dust inhalation. Devin was on steroids more often than not, and still he had asthma attacks.

After Devin had another severe attack at eighteen months of age, his mother brought him to us. "Although I was skeptical," she says, "I was willing to try anything that might help my little boy." After nine days on the Simplification Diet, Devin made a remarkable recovery. During the Challenge Phase, Devin's mother learned that he was allergic to six common foods. His parents decided to give up all medication and give the diet program an extended try.

At the next visit to the pediatrician, the doctor listened to Devin's lungs. He exclaimed that the steroids must finally be working because it was the first time he had heard no wheezing sounds. Devin's mother explained that although they had tried many approaches, only the Simplification Diet Program was successful. To this day, Devin continues to enjoy good health so long as he eats the right foods.

Despite many successful studies and case histories like these, the diagnosis and treatment of food allergies is still a controversial issue. As mentioned in chapter one, the field of medicine is by nature conservative and slow to accept "new" ideas. But studies like these underscore the relationship between our well-being and the foods we eat. In the future, we predict that you will see more and more medical doctors who recommend the Simplification Diet Program.

DO I HAVE FOOD ALLERGIES?

If you've been to a medical doctor and still have no explanation for your symptoms or have inadequate relief, prolonged complaints, or poor response to treatment, you are a likely candidate for the food allergy detection program presented here. By filling out the following questionnaire, you can begin to determine if your symptoms are likely to have been caused by an allergic reaction. Check either "yes" or "no" to each question.

QUESTIONNAIRE

	Yes	*No*
1. Do you have headaches more than once a month?	_____	_____
2. Do you have breathing problems during exercise?	_____	_____
3. Do you have an adverse reaction to chemical smells, cigarette smoke, or perfume?	_____	_____
4. Do you have a chronically stuffed or drippy nose?	_____	_____
5. Do you have itchy or watery eyes?	_____	_____
6. Do you have skin problems or itchy skin which may have been called eczema in some cases, or hives in others?	_____	_____
7. If you are a woman, do you have excessive vaginal discharge?	_____	_____

8. Do you have aches in your limbs or recurrent muscle spasms? _____ _____

9. Do you feel that you are unusually fatigued physically and/or depressed emotionally? _____ _____

10. Do you feel that your thinking is foggy and not sharply focused? _____ _____

11. Do you have stomach pains, or lots of gas particularly after meals? _____ _____

12. Do you have diarrhea or constipation (may be called irritable bowel syndrome)? _____ _____

13. Do you have painful, achy joints (also called arthritis)? _____ _____

14. Do you feel anxious and have a very quick temper? (In children this may be called hyperactive or hyperkinetic behavior.) _____ _____

15. Do you have hay fever or any other allergies? _____ _____

16. Are you sensitive to mold or mildew? Are your symptoms aggravated in damp, dark, or musty places? _____ _____

17. Does your pulse race or is your heartbeat irregular after eating? _____ _____

18. Does anyone in your family have hay fever or allergies to foods or inhalants? _____ _____

19. Do you experience infections of any type more than twice a year? _____ _____

20. Do you have, or have you ever had, seizures? _____ _____

If you answered yes to two or more of these questions, the Simplification Diet Program is probably for you. This questionnaire, however, serves only as a general base from which to start our exploration of your problem.

WHAT THE SIMPLIFICATION DIET PROGRAM INVOLVES

The Simplification Diet Program begins with the Simplification Phase. In this part of the program, your diet is simplified for one week by eliminating foods that research has shown are likely to cause allergic reactions. (A list of these foods is in chapter three.) In these seven days, your body will have a chance to clear itself of the residue of these commonly problematic foods and stop reacting adversely to them. You may notice a dramatic reduction or cessation of symptoms during this seven-day period.

After this Simplification Phase, you will begin the Challenge Phase in which the problem foods are reintroduced into your diet one by one at two-day intervals. During this phase, which may take as few as eighteen days, you'll keep a food diary to record any adverse reactions when a particular food is ingested. This is how you will pinpoint the foods to which your body reacts.

Once you have isolated your problem food(s), you will obviously want to learn how to live without them. The Simplification Diet Program will give you eating tips and recipes to help you incorporate other, nonreactive foods into your new diet, and teach you new healthy eating habits.

You will get the most benefit from the Simplification Diet Program if you are committed to making it work. You have the first step if you believe that food allergies are a health problem that can be successfully diagnosed and treated. And you have the chance to achieve a pain- and symptom-free life if you embrace this program and give it an honest try. If you can make the commitment, read on, because a healthier you may be only seven days away.

Read the following chapters very carefully before beginning the program. They take you step-by-step through each phase so you'll know exactly what you are doing, where you are going, and what to expect in the end.

3 · Step-by-Step through the Simplification Diet Program

STEP I
PLANNING AHEAD

We know you're anxious to find the cause of your food allergy, but you'll find the Simplification and Challenge phases of this program easier to follow if you've prepared yourself and your household in advance. Take some time before beginning the program to consider the nine suggestions that follow.

One: Notify Your Physician

Remember, if you are under a doctor's treatment or on prescription medication, contact your doctor. He or she may want to modify your medication schedule while you are on this diet because this diet often reduces the need for medication.

Two: Stop Taking Supplements and Reduce Your Caffeine Intake

During the Simplification Phase eliminate all vitamin and mineral supplements that you are currently taking. Because many B complex vitamins have a yeast base, and most vitamin fillers contain a corn ingredient, vitamins and supplements may contain one or more of your problem foods. However, if you take many daily supplements, it is not good to stop all of them "cold turkey," so cut down on their use gradually over the five- to ten-day period before you plan to begin the Simplification Phase. If you are currently taking only one or two supplements each day, you can stop them when you begin the diet program without any adverse effects.

If you are drinking more than three cups of coffee a day, it would be wise to reduce this by one cup a day until you are drinking only two cups the day before you begin the Simplification Diet Program. Immediately stopping a large caffeine intake (this includes large amounts of black tea or caffeinated soda) often brings about a splitting headache. To avoid this, slowly wean yourself from caffeine.

Three: Prepare Your Family and Friends

Before you begin the program, prepare your family and friends. Explain what you plan to do and ask for their support. If you have ever been on a reducing diet, you know how helpful it is to know that those near you support and encourage you.

It will also be easier for you if everyone in your household agrees to eat the foods prescribed on this diet when they eat at home. Not only does this show support, but it makes mealtime less of a cooking ordeal. And they may benefit as well!

Four: Stock Up

Before you begin eliminating any foods from your diet, go shopping and stock up on the foods you will be allowed to eat. The foods you can eat during the seven to fourteen days of the Simplification Phase are:

VEGETABLES

artichoke
asparagus
avocado
beets
bok choy
broccoli
brussels sprouts
cabbage
carrots
cauliflower
celery
chicory
collards
cucumbers
dandelion
eggplant
endive
escarole
horseradish (fresh, no vinegar)
kale
kohlrabi
legumes (black-eyed peas, kidney beans, lentils, lima beans, navy beans, peas, soybeans, string beans)
lettuce (leaf or head)
mustard greens
okra
onions
parsnips
peppers
potatoes (white, sweet, or yams)
pumpkin
radish
rutabaga
spinach
squash (winter or summer)
swiss chard
tomatoes
turnips
watercress

FRUIT

apples
apricots
bananas
blackberries
blueberries
cherries
coconut
cranberries
loganberries
melons (all, including cantaloupe, honeydew, watermelon)
nectarines
peaches
pears
persimmons
pineapple
plums
prunes
pomegranate
raspberries

MEATS AND SEAFOOD

beef*
chicken
clams
crab
duck
fish
game birds
goose
lamb*
lobster

oysters
pheasant
pork*
quail
rabbit
shrimp
squirrel
turkey
veal*
venison

FLOUR

amaranth flour
barley flour
millet flour
oat flour
potato flour
rice flour
rye flour

GRAINS

amaranth
barley
buckwheat (this is not wheat!)
millet
oats
brown rice
rye

SWEETENERS

barley malt
honey
pure maple syrup
rice syrup

HERBS AND SPICES

all, but fresh are preferable
to dried because they are
less likely to be moldy
(thus containing yeast)

OIL

olive
safflower
sesame
soy
sunflower
walnut

NUTS AND SEEDS

nuts: almonds, Brazil, cashews, filberts, hazelnuts,
pecans, walnuts (no pea-
nuts)
seeds: pumpkin, sesame,
sunflower

BEVERAGES

fresh vegetable juice†
herbal tea (without any citrus)
water (tap, bottled, or
seltzer)

*A maximum of two red meat meals per week is recommended.
†Avoid all commercial vegetable juices.

Five: Out of Sight, Out of Mind

Before beginning the Simplification Phase, go through the list of foods that will be eliminated from your diet (pages 39–42) and put them away. Push perishables to the back of the bottom shelf in your refrigerator, or give them away. Box up and store away all the others. Remember the old saying: "Out of Sight, Out of Mind."

Six: Record Present Symptoms

During the Simplification Phase, you will be watching to see if your symptoms lessen or cease. To assure yourself of accurate results, write down exactly how you feel during the week before you begin the program. Sometimes when symptoms stop, we forget they were ever a problem. It will be helpful if you can look back on a written record.

Seven: Weigh and Record

On the day before you begin the Simplification Diet Program, weigh yourself and note your weight. You will also weigh and record your weight every day during the program. Because some people retain water and get bloated and puffy in reaction to a particular food, it is very common to lose up to six pounds of water in the first two or three days of the Simplification Phase. You will not be losing fat or burning extra calories; you will simply be eliminating fluid. No one knows exactly why people with food allergies tend to retain fluid. But many people do report that they lose that bloated feeling after they have been avoiding foods to which they are allergic. So, on the day before you plan to begin the program, record your weight.

As you enter the Challenge Phase of the program a weight gain (sometimes as much as two or three pounds overnight) almost always indicates that you have reintroduced a food to which you are allergic. It will be important to have a record of your weight fluctuations.

Eight: Keep a Food Diary

Prepare a food diary. Buy yourself a notebook. Record all of your present symptoms on the first page, then set aside a separate page for each day of the entire program. When you begin the Simplification Diet Program, you'll be ready to keep a written record of how you feel each day, as well as your weight and food intake. Following the sample food diary printed below, you will record the date and your weight each morning. Then you will list all the foods you eat and note the time of day they are eaten. You will also record how you feel, and make note of any symptoms you may be having.

To identify your problem food, it is vital to have this written record. It is your only means of objectively monitoring your symptoms and documenting your improvements.

SAMPLE FOOD DIARY

Date _____

Morning Weight _____

Time	Food or Drink	Amount	Symptoms
8:00 A.M.	granola (wheat-free!)	½ cup	tired, irritable, didn't sleep well last night
	soy milk	¾ cup	
	herbal tea	1 cup	
11:00 A.M.	pear	1	
1:00 P.M.	grilled hamburger	4 oz.	fine, no symptoms
	rice cakes	2	
	carrot sticks	6	
	celery sticks	6	
4:00 P.M.	banana	1	
7:00 P.M.	baked chicken	2 breasts	
	green beans	½ cup	
	baked potato	1	
	soy margarine	1 T	
	brown rice	1 cup	
	almond cookies	4	

Nine: Set Your Goals

Most people work best when they have a goal to work toward. Think of something you've been wanting for a long time and promise it to yourself as a reward when you finish this program. Maybe you'd like some new clothes, a vacation, or a party. Whatever reward you choose, visualize yourself moving through the Simplification Diet Program well prepared, in good spirits, and ultimately attaining your goal.

STEP II
THE SIMPLIFICATION PHASE
(DAYS ONE TO SEVEN)

Now it's time to completely stop eating all the foods that commonly cause food sensitivities. The process is simple: from day one to day seven, you do not eat any of the foods listed on pages 39–42. Do not ease into this phase by eliminating some foods on one day and more on the next. Eliminate them all from your diet right from the start. You should notice a drastic reduction or total cessation of symptoms within seven days. Then you will start reintroducing these eliminated foods during the Challenge Phase. However, if there is no change in the way you feel after the first seven days on the Simplification Diet, you may be one of the few people whose body chemistry takes longer to recover from having eaten a problem food. If so, continue this Simplification Phase for an additional seven days before beginning the Challenge Phase.

The key to successfully simplifying your diet is to recognize the many components that make up a single food. Rye bread, for example, may appear to be an "O.K." food because rye flour is permissible, but packaged rye bread usually contains wheat flour as well as rye flour. Since wheat products must be eliminated, rye bread is also out. Because of combined ingredients, many foods join the elimination list. Ketchup may seem fine because tomatoes are allowed, but it also contains the eliminated ingredient vinegar. White rice sounds O.K., but it is usually enriched, which means that B vitamins have been added. Since they are often derived from yeast, it's out. Salad dressings, luncheon meats, soups, pastries, pickles, and sauerkraut are all forbidden because of their other ingredients. From this short list of examples, you can see the importance of considering the components that make up the foods you eat during the Simplification Phase. As a general rule, all processed and packaged foods should be avoided because they almost always contain something that is eliminated on this diet. Therefore, it is easiest during this period of simplification to use single, fresh ingredients.

Another way to make sure you're not eating things that should be eliminated is to read all food ingredient labels. You will be most successful during this phase if you do not eat anything unless you know what it's made of. Sometimes, labels list ingredients by their chemical or by-product names. Words that mean "sugar," for example, end in -ose, such as glucose, sucrose, fructose, or dextrose. These are included on the list of eliminated foods.

We have also included a list of "forbidden" foods, but it is impossible to include every item available in every food category. So remember: read all labels carefully.

At this point, you should have your shelves stocked with the foods that are allowed on this diet (pages 34–35), and now it's time to eliminate the following foods.

CITRUS

Eliminate all citrus foods:
grapefruit
lemons
limes
oranges
citrus beverages

CHOCOLATE AND COLA

Eliminate all chocolate and
   cola:
cakes
candies
chocolate cereals
chocolate and cola drinks
frosting

pastries
pies

COFFEE, TEA, AND ALCOHOL

Eliminate all coffee and tea
   (regular or decaffeinated),
   and alcohol, including beer
   and wine. Remember to
   reduce coffee intake
   slowly.

CORN

Eliminate all corn and foods
   that contain corn products:
bacon
candies

corn batters
corn breads
corn chips
corn flakes
other corn-containing cereals
corn muffins
corn starches
corn syrups
dextrin
dextrose
envelope and stamp adhesive
fresh and frozen corn
fructose
hominy grits
ketchup
maize
Mazola oil
mixed vegetable oil
modified food starch
peanut butter with corn syrup
popcorn
toothpaste
tortillas
zein

DAIRY

Eliminate all dairy products
and foods that may con-
tain dairy ingredients:
butter
biscuits
cookies
cottage cheese
crackers
cream soups
doughnuts
ice cream
luncheon meats
milk (whole, skim, evapo-
rated, goat's, condensed,
instant nonfat dry)

pastries
yogurt
Read labels for milk-derived
ingredients such as casein,
lactoalbumin, and whey.

EGGS

Eliminate all eggs and foods
that contain egg products:
bread
cakes (including all cake
mixes)
cookies
custard
eggs in any form (poached,
scrambled, baked, fried,
creamed, deviled, hard- or
soft-boiled)
egg salad
egg sauces
ice cream
mayonnaise
meringues
noodles
omelets
pasta
pies
prepared mixes and frozen
dinners
salad dressings
soufflés
Read labels for egg-derived
ingredient albumin.

SUGAR

Eliminate all sugar and
sugar products (including
brown sugar). The list of
foods that contain sugar
is far too extensive to
print. Avoid all the ob-
vious sugar foods such as

candy, cake, and soft drinks. Read labels for words that end in -ose, such as glucose, sucrose, fructose, or dextrose.

VITAMINS AND MINERALS

Taper off your use of supplements in a 5–10 day period before beginning the Simplification Phase. Then, when you begin the program, eliminate all vitamins and minerals.

WHEAT

Eliminate all wheat and foods that contain wheat products:
biscuits
bran
bread (wheat, white, rye, pumpernickel)
bulgur
commercial gravy
cookies
cous-cous
crackers
doughnuts
farina
flour (wheat, graham, white, high gluten, enriched, unbleached)
French toast
matzos
meats containing fillers (meat loaf, weiners, bologna, luncheon meats)
muffins
noodles
pancakes
pastries
prepared batters and mixes
rolls
semolina
soups (with noodles, dumplings, or thickened with wheat flour)
soy sauce
tabouli
wheat cereals
wheat germ

YEAST

Eliminate all yeast and foods which contain or are made from yeast:
baker's yeast
brewer's yeast
condiments that contain vinegar (mustard, ketchup, relish, horseradish, pickles, mayonnaise)
dried fruits
fermented foods (miso soup, soy sauce)
grapes
nutritional yeast
peanuts
sauerkraut
vinegar

ARTIFICIAL COLORINGS

Eliminate all artificial colorings. Yellow dye no. 5 (tartrazine) is especially problematic. It is found in:
butterscotch chips
cake mixes
candy drops and hard candies

certain breakfast cereals
certain candy coatings
certain ice creams and sherbets
certain instant and regular puddings
colored marshmallows
chocolate chips
commercial frostings
commercial gingerbread
commercial pies
flavored carbonated beverages
flavored drink mixes
ready-to-eat canned puddings
refrigerated rolls and quick breads

ARTIFICIAL FLAVORINGS

Eliminate all artificial flavorings.

ARTIFICIAL PRESERVATIVES

Eliminate all artificial preservatives including: sodium benzoate (also called benzoic acid)
BHA
BHT

ARTIFICIAL SWEETENERS

Eliminate all artificial sweeteners:
aspartame
NutraSweet
saccharine

SEASONINGS

Don't pick up anything and shake it on your food until you read the label.

That's the entire list! Once you've decided to eliminate these foods from your diet, stick with it. While you're in the Simplification Phase, you must be very strict about avoiding these foods because it simply won't work if you say to yourself, "Oh, a little bit won't make a difference." The tiniest morsel certainly will make a difference—it could compromise the whole program.

It's not really difficult to get by without these foods for such a short period of time, especially when there are others you can substitute in their place. (See chapter four for substitutions and recipes.)

STEP III
THE CHALLENGE PHASE
(DAYS EIGHT THROUGH TWENTY-FIVE)

It is time to reintroduce to your diet the foods that were eliminated during the Simplification Phase, and watch to see which ones cause an allergic reaction. This part of the program is called the Challenge Phase because you're challenging your system to react to commonly problematic foods. If there is no adverse reaction, your body has met the challenge and has proved it can handle the reintroduced food. If there is an adverse reaction, however, you have identified one of your problem foods.

It would be too confusing to reintroduce all the foods at one time and then try to figure out which one caused your reaction. So the foods are allowed back into your diet one food group at a time at two-day intervals. There are nine food groups, so this phase will take eighteen days. As each food group is reintroduced, the foods must be eaten in large quantities. Just a small nibble won't necessarily cause a reaction. To be absolutely sure of detecting food sensitivities, you need to eat a reasonably large amount of the suspect foods each day for two full days. The best way to ensure a good amount is to have a serving of the reintroduced food at each meal. The suggested menus for each food group that are included in this chapter will help you do this.

If you do have a reaction to one of the foods during this phase, do not continue eating that food or reintroducing any additional foods until the symptoms totally cease. For example, if you reintroduce corn and citrus with no problems and then reintroduce eggs and have a reaction, stop eating eggs and egg products for however long it takes to become unreactive. The time period for this to occur varies. It can be as short as one day or as long as a week to ten days, depending on your system. Don't worry about it, though. You have discovered one of your problem foods; that's the goal of this phase. Continue eating all the foods that you were allowed on the Simplification Diet, as well as the foods that were reintroduced without a reaction, until you feel well again. Then reintroduce the next food on the list, completely eliminating the food group that caused your reaction.

If your symptoms do not recur upon the reintroduction of a particular food during the two days, you can simply continue eating that food in regular-size servings whenever you wish and go on to the next group on the list. Since you have been able to eat successfully large quantities of a given food for two days in a row without any reaction, you can safely assume you are not allergic to it.

Before you begin this phase, remember to:

- read through the list of food suggestions in advance and stock up
- continue to read food labels. During this phase it is still best to stay away from processed and packaged foods because they usually contain a combination of many ingredients. Do not reintroduce any food that contains a problem ingredient that has not yet been reintroduced.
- introduce only one food group at a time
- continue eating the foods allowed during the Simplification Phase
- record each day's food, weight, and symptom information in your food diary.

The following food groups are to be reintroduced in the order in which they are listed. The suggested food and menu ideas are not mandatory; they are only included as a guide to help you. The asterisk (*) after an item indicates that a recipe for it is found in chapter four.

Reintroduce the food groups in this order:

1. Corn
2. Citrus
3. Eggs
4. Yeast-free wheat
5. Yeasted wheat
6. Yeast-free dairy products
7. Yeasted dairy products
8. Sugar
9. Coffee, tea

Days One and Two: Reintroduce Corn
Suggested Foods

Cornmeal Mush*
Quick Corn Bread*
corn tortillas (from health food store only)
100% corn noodles (available at health food stores)
fresh corn
frozen corn
hominy grits (unenriched)

Corn flakes (from a health food store only—others are often fortified with yeast-derived vitamins)

Suggested Menus

Breakfast: corn flakes (one bowl)
soy or nut milk
apple juice and/or a banana

Lunch: chef's salad with lettuce, raw vegetables, tuna fish and sub-stitution dressing of choice*
2 slices Quick Corn Bread* with soy margarine
potato salad with a substitution dressing*

Dinner: Mexican Beans with Enchilada Sauce*
2 to 3 corn tortillas
chopped cabbage with a substitution dressing*
steamed broccoli

Days Three and Four: Reintroduce Citrus
Suggested Foods

grapefruits
lemons or limes
oranges

Suggested Menus

Breakfast: oatmeal or corn flakes (if you had no reaction to corn)
soy or nut milk
½ cup orange juice or one orange

Lunch: large fruit salad including oranges or grapefruits (at least 1 orange or ½ grapefruit)
or 1 whole orange or grapefruit
nuts and other seasonal fruit
Wasa Lite Rye Crackers

Dinner: hamburger(s) or Sunny Burger(s)*
baked potato with soy margarine
steamed green beans with slivered roasted almonds
tossed salad with substitution dressing of choice*
broiled grapefruit half with honey or 1 orange

Days Five and Six: Reintroduce Eggs
Food Suggestions

cooked eggs (poached, hard- or soft-boiled, fried in olive oil)

Menu Suggestions

Breakfast: oatmeal with 2 poached eggs on top
or 2 eggs any style with Wasa Lite Rye Crackers
herbal tea or orange juice (if you had no reaction to citrus)

Lunch: egg salad made with substitution dressing of choice*
rice cakes or Wasa Lite Rye Crackers
raw vegetable sticks
potato salad made with substitution dressing of choice*

Dinner: two-egg omelet
vegetable of choice
Brown Rice with Sesame Seasoning*
salad with substitution dressing*

Days Seven and Eight: Reintroduce Yeast-free Wheat

On the list of food groups to be reintroduced during this Challenge
Phase, you'll notice that the wheat and dairy categories are divided
into "yeast-free" and "yeasted" sections. Because yeast and wheat
are each a possible cause of food sensitivity, they must be reintroduced separately. The reason for this is that if you were to reintroduce all the foods from the wheat group listed in the Simplification
Phase and then had an adverse reaction, you would not know if
the problem was caused by the wheat or by the yeast in the wheat
foods.

Food Suggestions

bulgur
chapatti (a wheat tortilla found in health food stores)
Blueberry Pancakes*
Blueberry* or Pumpkin Nut* muffins
pasta (unenriched, available at health food stores)
Cranberry Bread*

Menu Suggestions

Breakfast: Blueberry Pancakes* or Cranberry Bread* (at least 2 pancakes or 2 slices of the bread)
1 egg, and/or orange juice (if you had no reactions when reintroduced)

Lunch: tossed salad with substitution dressing*
Three Bean Salad*
1–2 Blueberry Muffins*
piece of fruit

Dinner: 1 cup pasta
spaghetti sauce (homemade; if not, read the label carefully)
or meat, fish, or chicken with baked potato
steamed spinach or asparagus
cucumber salad with substitution dressing of choice*
1–2 slices of Cranberry Bread*

Days Nine and Ten: Reintroduce Yeasted Wheat
Food Suggestions

bread
crackers

Make sure you read all labels to ensure they do not include other ingredients you know you are allergic to, or that you have not yet reintroduced.

Menu Suggestions

Breakfast: 2 slices of whole wheat toast (read the label carefully)
cereal of choice (read the label carefully) or eggs (if you had no reaction)
soy or nut milk

Lunch: Chicken Salad Platter* with 2 slices whole wheat bread
tossed salad

Dinner: fish of choice
Vegetable Barley Soup*
5–8 three-inch-square wheat crackers
steamed cauliflower
steamed string beans

Days Eleven and Twelve:
Reintroduce Yeast-free Dairy Products
Food Suggestions

butter
cottage cheese (additive-free)
farmer's cheese
milk
plain yogurt
ricotta cheese

Menu Suggestions

Breakfast: cereal of choice with ½ cup milk
fruit or juice
toast with butter

Lunch: fruit salad with ½ cup yogurt or ½ cup cottage cheese

Dinner: chicken (broiled or baked)
baked potato with butter
vegetable of choice
salad with substitution dressing of choice* (you may use vinegar if
    you have no reaction to yeast)
unsweetened canned pineapple with scoop of ricotta cheese
½ cup milk

Days Thirteen and Fourteen:
Reintroduce Yeasted Dairy Products
Food Suggestions

hard cheese such as cheddar, mozzarella, jarlsburg, and swiss lor-
    raine (do not use processed cheese or those with orange color)

Menu Suggestions

Breakfast: cheese omelet
rice cakes or Wasa Lite Rye Crackers with 2 slices (minimum) cheese
    broiled on top

Lunch: tossed salad with at least 6 one-inch-square chunks of cheese
crackers of choice

Dinner: Light and Lovely Split Pea Soup*
lamb chops
mashed potatoes with chives and 2 slices of melted cheese
steamed green beans
tossed salad

Days Fifteen and Sixteen: Reintroduce Sugar

Consume a minimum of 5 sugar cubes at each meal, or use 3–5
teaspoons of sugar sprinkled on foods eaten for dessert at each
meal.

Days 17 and 18: Reintroduce Coffee and/or Tea

Go back to the number of cups of coffee or other caffeinated beverages you were drinking per day before you began the Simplification Diet Program.

If you felt an immediate adverse reaction to a reintroduced food,
your job of detection was easy, and your food allergy was quickly
uncovered. But because some food allergies cause delayed reactions, you may need to carefully study your food diary to accurately
relate the symptom to the food.

When you have found your problem food(s), the battle is half
won. But now it's up to you to adjust your diet around these foods.
Chapter four will help you do that. It is full of diet tips, menu
ideas, and recipes.

While you're learning to live without some of the processed and
packaged foods you're used to, you may worry that you're spending
too much time in the kitchen preparing foods from scratch. This
may be true in the beginning but remember, when you spend more
time in the kitchen, you spend less time in a sickbed, absent from
work, or missing life's good times. So bring out the good food and
embrace your new life with joy. Your simplification diet isn't a ball

and chain, it is the key to years of good health. It also doesn't forbid you from ever again tasting the foods you love.

When Marie discovered that she was sensitive to sugar, she felt the whole program had been a waste of time because she knew she could never stay away from all the chocolate goodies she loved. But her tears disappeared when we told her the good news about food allergies: if you abstain from your problem food for a while, it can usually be brought back into your diet on a limited basis without any adverse reaction. Only when the food is eaten in excess of your tolerance level will you react negatively to an "overdose."

We can't tell you exactly how long you must abstain from a problem food before your body will be ready to accept small amounts again. Nor can we predict how often you will be able to eat a problem food without a reaction. Everyone's body chemistry is so unique that only personal experimentation will give you those answers.

Marie waited two months before she tried a small piece of chocolate. She was delighted to see that her nausea and headaches did not return. She continued to eat a small piece each day until, on the third day, her symptoms attacked with full force. But this time Marie was not worried or upset because she knew what the problem was and she knew how to stop it. She was now in control of her own health.

So wait a while; let your body chemistry readjust, then challenge your system again by giving your problem food another try.

4 · Cooking Tips, Recipes, and Menu Ideas

In this chapter, you will find food preparation tips, food substitution recipes, breakfast, lunch, and dinner recipes, and dinner menu ideas. There are also recipes to help you through the Challenge Phase. All of this information is given as a help and a guide. None of it is mandatory. You can use our suggestions or combine the foods on the allowed foods list to create your own meal plans. There is a blank meal plan schedule at the end of this chapter to help you do this. Whether you choose to follow our food plan or make up your own, you will soon find that the Simplification Diet Program allows you plenty of foods to eat and enjoy!

PREPARATION TIPS

Steam Cooking. It is always best to steam rather than boil your vegetables because many nutrients are water soluble and are lost when cooked in water. You won't lose these nutrients or any of the flavor when you steam cook. To do it, just chop the vegetables, place them on a steamer tray over boiling water, and steam just until tender.
Morning Soaking. Before you leave the house in the morning, get beans and/or grain soaking in the pots in which they will be cooked. This speeds up your cooking time later. It also allows for the bean or grain to begin to sprout, thus transforming the minerals in these foods into a form that is more easily absorbed.

Think Big. When cooking brown rice or any whole grain, cook a large enough amount for use throughout the week (i.e., for making breakfasts, stir-fry meals, rice balls, rice pudding, and so on). You can also prepare large batches of beans or meat and use them in dinner recipes and as leftovers throughout the week.

These cooking charts will help you prepare these foods.

COOKING GRAINS

One Cup Grain	Cooking Water	Regular Cooking Time	Pressure Cooking Water	Pressure Cooking Time	Yield
Barley	2½ c.	1¼ hours	2½ c.	1 hour	3 c.
Brown rice	2 c.	1 hour (for fluffy American style)	1¼ c.	45 min. (for heartier and stickier Oriental rice)	3 c.
Buckwheat groats	2 c.	20 min.	2 c.	10 min.	2 c.
Bulgur	1¾ c.	15 min.	1¾ c.	10 min.	2½ c.
Cornmeal	3 c.	30 min.	——	——	4 c.
Millet	3 c.	40 min.	2¾ c.	15 min.	3½ c.
Rolled oats	3 c.	15 min.	——	——	3 c.
Whole oats	3 c.	1½ hours	2 c.	1¼ hours	3 c.
Whole wheat berries	3½ c.	2½ hours	3 c.	1½ hours	3 c.

COOKING LEGUMES

One Cup Legumes	Cooking Water	Regular Cooking Time	Pressure Cooking Time	Yield
Aduki beans	4 c.	1¾ hours	45 min.	3 c.
Black beans	3 c.	2 hours	20–25 min.	2¼ c.
Black-eyed peas	3 c.	1 hour	30–35 min.	2¼ c.
Chick peas (garbanzo beans)	6 c.	3–4 hours	1 hour 15 min.	3 c.
Kidney beans	4 c.	1¾ hours	45 min.	2¼ c.
Lentils	3 c.	45 mins.	10–15 min.	3 c.
Lima beans	4 c.	1¾ hours	35 min.	2¼ c.
Mung beans	4 c.	1 hour	30–35 min.	3 c.
Navy beans	3 c.	1 hour	30–35 min.	2¼ c.
Pinto beans	3 c.	2½ hours	40–45 min.	2¼ c.
Split peas	3 c.	45 min.	10–15 min.	3 c.
Soy beans	4 c.	4–5 hours	2 hours	2½ c.

After sorting for stones and rinsing soak 1 cup of beans in 3 cups water for 8 hours (optional). Do not soak lentils or split peas.

Boiling Method
1. Pour off soaking water.
2. Add fresh water, cover, and bring to a boil.
3. Boil beans for ten minutes with lid off.
4. Skim the foam from top of the beans. (This seems to make them easier to digest. You can skip this step if you choose.)
5. Cover and cook at medium heat, referring to chart for time.

Crockpot Method
Best done first thing in the morning.

1. Get a pot of water boiling.
2. Sort and rinse beans.
3. Put beans in crockpot and add appropriate amount of *boiling* water (beans *must* boil at some point in order to get soft).
4. Turn crockpot to low; beans may now be left unattended.
5. Beans are done anywhere from two to six hours, depending on the bean.
6. Drain beans, saving the liquid for a soup base.

When using a crockpot, don't worry if the beans cook longer than you planned—on low they will not burn. They are simply ready when you are!

Pressure-cooking Method

Follow the same steps as for the boiling method. Adjust heat once you have reached pressure so that the weight on the pressure cooker bobbles gently for the duration of the cooking time.

Beans can be used as part of a recipe, or simply sautéed with olive oil, onions, garlic, and a pinch of salt. Delicious!

SUBSTITUTION RECIPES

Here are substitutions and recipes for some of your favorite foods that contain an eliminated ingredient:

1. *Baking Powder.* In place of your regular baking powder, use corn-free baking powder which you can buy or order at a health food store, or mix together the following ingredients and store in a jar.

1 teaspoon cream of tartar
1 teaspoon arrowroot
½ teaspoon baking soda

2. *Bread.*

- Wasa Lite Rye Crackers
- Kavli Norwegian Crispbread, Thin Style
- rice cakes
- Rye Flour Tortillas (see p. 91)
- 100% Plus Rye Bread by Dimpflmeier Bakery, Ltd.

If your health food store doesn't carry this bread, they can order it from:

Dimpflmeier Bakery, Ltd.
33 Advance Road
Toronto, Ontario, Canada
M8Z 2T4
800–268–2421

Dimpflmeier uses a new sourdough culture derived from bacteria (not yeast) every week. They have it specially made for them in Germany. Do not assume that you can buy any other brand of sourdough bread, because most sourdough cultures are used over and over again and usually pick up wild yeasts during the process.

- Brown Rice Snaps

These are delicious, crunchy crackers made from brown rice and can be purchased at a health food store. Read the ingredients label and purchase the plain or sesame seed variety. Avoid the ones made with tamari as this is a soy sauce and contains yeast and wheat.

3. *Butter.* Although margarine is not a healthy food to eat in general, for the Simplification Phase it is an allowable substitute for butter. Buy 100 percent soy margarine at a health food store or make sure you buy one that is corn- and dairy- (whey) free at the supermarket.

4. *Coffee.* Look for Roma coffee substitute by Natural Touch (in health food stores).

5. *Eggs*. You cannot eat cooked or raw eggs, or any of the commercial egg substitutes (such as Egg Beaters). But if you need an egg as a binding ingredient in a recipe, you can substitute the following egg equivalents:

- Dissolve one package of unflavored gelatin in boiling water. Use 2–3 tablespoons of this liquid instead of one egg.
- One teaspoon of arrowroot (which you can buy at health food stores) equals one egg.
- Ener-G Egg Replacer is a powder that can be found at health food stores. Use 1 teaspoon Ener-G Egg Replacer in 2 tablespoons water to equal one egg.

6. *Flour*. In place of one cup flour (white or whole wheat) called for in a recipe, use any of the following:

- one cup rye flour
- a combination of ½ cup rye flour with ½ cup oat flour (to make oat flour, blend old-fashioned or quick rolled oats in a blender, or buy oat flour at a health food store)
- a mixture of ½ cup rye flour with ½ cup skinned, cooked (baked or boiled) mashed potato (white or sweet potato)
- a combination of ¼ cup ground nuts with ¾ cup skinned, cooked (baked or boiled) mashed potato
- a mixture of ½ cup oat flour plus ½ cup rice flour (available at health food stores).

7. *Ketchup*. All commercial ketchups contain vinegar and should not be used. A delicious substitute can be found in the recipe for Sunny Burgers with Tomato Sauce, p. 84.

8. *Mayonnaise*. Make one or both of these delicious "mayonnaise" recipes.

AVOCADO MAYONNAISE

        1   avocado, peeled and pitted
        1   cup olive oil
    1–2   garlic cloves
        1   teaspoon chopped onion
        1   teaspoon curry powder

Blend all ingredients together in a blender at high speed. Chill. *Makes 1¹/₂ cups.*

WALNUT MAYONNAISE

      1 cup walnuts or unroasted cashews
    ³/₄ cup olive oil
      2 teaspoons chopped onion
    ¹/₂ teaspoon salt
      1 teaspoon powdered dry mustard
         water or chicken broth (optional; see p. 67)

Place walnuts or cashews in blender at high speed until finely chopped. Reduce speed and slowly add olive oil. Blend well. Add onion, salt, and mustard to mixture. Blend well. Add water or chicken broth, if necessary, to achieve a creamy consistency. Chill. *Makes 1¹/₂ cups.*

9. *Milk.* In place of any kind of milk (whole, skim, low fat, evaporated, condensed, instant nonfat dry) use the following substitutions.

NUT MILK

    ³/₄ cup raw almonds
    3¹/₂ cups water
      2 tablespoons honey
         dash alcohol-free vanilla extract (see p. 60)

In a blender, blend almonds at high speed until they form a uniform powder (it may help to turn the blender on and off several times). Fill the blender with water. Add honey and vanilla. Blend for 30 seconds. Store in a jar in the refrigerator; it will keep for 5–7 days. *Makes one quart.*

■ You can buy soy milk at a health food store, but make sure that the brand names are Health Valley Soy Moo, Sunsoy, or Soy M; if not, read the ingredients. Many brands of soy milk contain corn oil. Soy milk powder is also available.

10. *Mustard.* Instead of using commercially prepared mustard, which contains vinegar, use the following recipe to make your own.

HOMEMADE MUSTARD

> 2–3 tablespoons water
> ¼ cup powdered mustard
> 2 tablespoons olive oil (optional)

Stir water and powdered mustard together to make a paste. Store in a closed jar in the refrigerator. If the mixture is too hot for your taste, you can tone it down with olive oil. *Makes ¼ cup.*

11. *Salad Dressing.* To avoid commercially prepared salad dressing, these substitutions are delicious and easy to make.

AVOCADO DRESSING

> 2 avocados, peeled and pitted
> ½ cup honey
> ½ cup sunflower oil
> ½ teaspoon ground nutmeg
>   dash salt and/or water, if needed

Place avocados in a blender with honey, sunflower oil, nutmeg, and salt. Blend well. If the avocados are dry, you may need to add a touch of water to make the mixture creamy.

MUSTARD ITALIAN DRESSING

> 1 cup olive oil
> ⅓ cup water
> 1 teaspoon dry mustard powder
> ⅓ teaspoon salt
> 1 tablespoon dried basil
> ½ teaspoon garlic powder (optional)
> ½ teaspoon onion powder (optional)

Blend all ingredients and store in a closed jar in the refrigerator. *Makes about 1½ cups.*

SALAD DRESSING À LA TOMATE

    1 cup olive oil
    ⅓ cup tomato juice, V-8 juice, or one fresh tomato
    ½ avocado, crushed (optional)
    ⅓ bunch watercress, chopped (optional)
    ½ small oñion, chopped (optional)
    1 tablespoon dried basil (optional)

Blend all ingredients and store in a closed jar in the refrigerator. *Makes about 1½ cups.*

12. *Sesame Seasonings.*

SESAME SALT

  sesame seeds
  salt

Roast some sesame seeds in the oven until they have a toasted flavor. In a blender, add ten parts sesame seeds to one part salt and blend until powdered. Store in a closed jar in a cool dark place. (This is great sprinkled on brown rice and/or vegetables.)

    Sesame seeds can be used as a flavorful topping for many foods. To toast, first rinse the seeds. Toast in frying pan or oven at medium heat, stirring every few minutes for 10 minutes or until golden brown and dry.

13. *Vanilla.* Pure alcohol-free vanilla extract can be found at health food stores. If your store does not carry it, ask them to order Spicery Shoppe Alcohol Free Vanilla Extract from:

Flavorchem Corporation
Downer's Grove, Illinois 60515
312–932–8100

HOMEMADE ALCOHOL-FREE VANILLA EXTRACT

    1 cup water
    2 vanilla beans

Place water and vanilla beans in uncovered saucepan. Bring to boil and continue to boil until liquid is reduced to ¼ cup. Strain and store in small, closed bottle in refrigerator.

Use these tasty substitutions in the many easy-to-prepare meals in this chapter and you'll see how easy it is to successfully complete the Simplification Diet Program.

BREAKFAST, LUNCH, AND DINNER RECIPES FOR THE SIMPLIFICATION PHASE
Breakfast Recipes

- Almond Crunch Granola
- Almond Fruit Shake
- Blueberry Pancakes
- Buckwheat Banana Muffins
- Buckwheat Pancakes
- Cold Cereal
- Continental Special
- Cream of Brown Rice
- Cream of Rye
- Hot Oat Bran Cereal
- Millet Potage
- Muesli
- Oatmeal
- Scrambled Tofu with Home Fries

ALMOND CRUNCH GRANOLA

    ¼ cup sesame oil
    ¼ cup maple syrup or honey
    1 teaspoon cinnamon (optional)

½ teaspoon alcohol-free vanilla extract (see p. 60; optional)
6 cups rolled oats
½ cup chopped almonds

Preheat oven to 300°F. Mix the oil and maple syrup or honey together. (Cinnamon and vanilla extract can be added to this mixture to taste, if desired.) Stir in the oats and almonds. Bake on cookie sheets until golden and crisp (approximately 25–30 minutes). Let cool and store in a closed jar in a dark, cool place. *Makes about 7 cups.*

ALMOND FRUIT SHAKE

12 almonds
1 cup water
1 teaspoon honey
1–2 pieces fruit

Soak the almonds in one cup of water overnight. Combine the soaked almonds and water in a blender until creamy. Add the honey and fruit (fruit ideas: apples, strawberries, bananas, peaches, apricots, or a handful of blueberries or raspberries). Blend well. *Serves 1.*

BLUEBERRY PANCAKES

2 cups rice flour
1 cup oat flour
1½ teaspoons baking soda
1 teaspoon salt
2 egg equivalents (see p. 56)
1 teaspoon olive or sesame oil
2½ cups water or Nut Milk (see p. 57)
1 cup blueberries (fresh or frozen, no sugar added)
olive oil for frying

Mix all ingredients in order given. Fry in olive oil until golden brown. Serve with commercial or homemade unsweetened applesauce (see p. 101). *Makes 12 pancakes.*

BUCKWHEAT BANANA MUFFINS

>   olive oil (for greasing muffin tin)
> 3/4 cups oat flour
> 1/2 cup buckwheat flour
> 2/3 teaspoon baking soda
> 1/8 teaspoon salt
> 1/4 cup sesame or safflower oil
> 1/4 cup honey
> 1   cup mashed ripe bananas

Preheat oven to 350°F. Oil muffin tin. Mix dry ingredients together in bowl. In another bowl, mix oil, honey, and mashed banana, then add this mixture to dry mixture. Stir. Fill muffin tins three-quarters full. Bake 20–30 minutes until golden brown. *Makes 12 muffins.*

BUCKWHEAT PANCAKES

>   1   cup buckwheat flour
>   1/2   cup brown rice flour
>   1/2   teaspoon baking soda
>   1 1/2 cups soy milk or Nut Milk (see p. 57)
>   4   tablespoons sesame oil
>   2   egg equivalents (see p. 56)
> 1/3–1/2 cup water (approximately)
>   olive oil for frying

Combine the flours and the baking soda. In a separate bowl, beat nut or soy milk, oil, and egg equivalents. Add this mixture to the dry, combining them well with quick strokes. Add water until you have a fairly runny batter. Fry in oiled skillet until brown on each side. *Makes about 2 dozen.*

COLD CEREAL

Serve one of the cereals (available at health food stores only) listed below with soy milk or Nut Milk (see p. 57).

- Oatio's by New Morning (read label—there are two kinds of Oatio's, one with wheat flour and one without)
- Crispy Brown Rice by Stow Mills or Erewhon.

CONTINENTAL SPECIAL

Toast a few slices of 100% Plus Rye Bread (see p. 55); spread with soy margarine and a 100% fruit jam of your choice.

CREAM OF BROWN RICE

    1 cup leftover brown rice
   ⅓ cup water, soy milk or Nut Milk (see p. 57)

Heat rice in water, Nut Milk, or soy milk to boiling. Pour into blender and blend until smooth. Serve plain or with Nut Milk or soy milk. Cream of Brown Rice can also be purchased at a health food store.

Note: *All white rice* is enriched with yeast-derived B vitamins and *cannot be used.*

CREAM OF RYE

Purchase Cream of Rye cereal from a health food store and follow directions on box.

HOT OAT BRAN CEREAL

Purchase Mother's Oat Bran cereal from a health food store and follow directions on box.

MILLET POTAGE

      1 cup millet
   3–4 cups water
         pinch salt
      2 tablespoons toasted chopped nuts or sesame seeds (op-
         tional; see p. 59)
      1 tablespoon tahini (optional)

Roast millet in a dry pan over medium heat. Grind millet in a blender. Place millet, water, and salt in saucepan. (The more water, the soupier the cereal.) Bring to a boil, cover, and simmer 15–20 minutes over low heat. Serve topped with toasted nuts or toasted, ground sesame seeds. For variety, stir in tahini when the millet is done. *Serves 4.*

MUESLI
A SWISS SPECIALTY

1 cup oat flakes (rolled oats), old-fashioned or quick, *not* instant
¼ cup coconut, shredded
¼ cup almonds, chopped
¼ cup sunflower seeds
¼ cup filberts, chopped
   water
   soy milk or Nut Milk (see p. 57)
¼ cup grated apples or chopped fresh fruit of the season

The night before, mix together in a bowl the oats, coconut, almonds, sunflower seeds, and filberts. Add just enough water to cover the mixture. Cover and place in refrigerator overnight to soften. Serve the next morning with soy milk or Nut Milk topped with grated apples or fruit of choice. *Serves 2.*

OATMEAL

½ cup rolled oats (old-fashioned, quick, or type available at health food store)
1¼ cups water, soy milk, or Nut Milk (see p. 57)
   pinch salt
⅛ cup chopped, roasted nuts (optional)
¼ cup unsweetened or homemade applesauce (optional; see p. 101)

Mix oats, water, and salt in saucepan. Cover and bring to a boil. Simmer for 10–20 minutes until soft. Serve oatmeal as is or add chopped, roasted nuts (except peanuts) and/or unsweetened applesauce. *Serves 2.*

SCRAMBLED TOFU WITH HOME FRIES

⅔ cup chopped scallions (2 medium-size)
⅓ cup chopped red pepper
1½ tablespoons olive oil

1 pound firm tofu, cut in small cubes
¼ cup chopped fresh parsley
⅓ teaspoon salt
¼ teaspoon ground marjoram
¼ teaspoon turmeric
    pinch cayenne pepper

Sauté the scallions and red peppers in olive oil over low heat in a large skillet. Add the tofu, parsley, salt, marjoram, and turmeric. Scramble gently until warm and well mixed (3–4 minutes). Add pinch of cayenne pepper. *Serves 2.*

Home Fries
Cube cooked potatoes and sauté in olive oil until brown. Add salt if desired.

Lunch Recipes

- Caesar's Leftovers
- Chicken Salad in a Curried Ring
- Chicken Salad Platter
- Fish Chowder
- Fruit Soup and Green Goddess Fruit Salad
- Hamburger with Tossed Salad
- Not Dogs
- Quick Lunches
- Rice Balls
- Shrimp Salad with Cream of Broccoli Soup
- Tofu Salad with Quick Creamed Carrot Soup
- Tuna Salad Bowl
- Veggie Burgers

CAESAR'S LEFTOVERS

One of the most efficient ways to move through the seven-day Simplification Phase is to use leftovers from dinner for lunch the next day. Cook extras of everything at dinner and place all the leftovers into one leak-proof covered plastic container. Your next meal, for instance, can combine diced chicken, steamed green beans, brown rice, and green salad. Dribble salad dressing of choice (see substitution recipes) down one side of container. Do *not* toss. Cover and refrigerate. Your lunch is then thoroughly chilled by morning when you are ready to take it to work. The food inside will keep cool at room temperature until lunchtime. Open container, toss, and eat.

CHICKEN SALAD IN A CURRIED RING

Curried Ring
       2 envelopes plain gelatin
    3⅓ cups chicken broth (see below)
       1 tablespoon curry powder
       1 cup Walnut Mayonnaise (see p. 57)
       2 tablespoons finely chopped onion
     ½ teaspoon salt
     ¼ teaspoon black pepper
       1 cup thinly sliced celery

Chicken Salad
       2 cups cubed chicken breast
     ½ cup Walnut Mayonnaise (see p. 57)
     ½ cup chopped celery

Accompaniments
       1 head ruby-leaf lettuce
       1 can water-packed black olives
            crackers (see p. 55)

Prepare curried ring in advance, allowing 4–5 hours to chill. Soften gelatin in 1 cup chicken broth for five minutes. Add curry powder and heat until mixture simmers and gelatin dissolves. Remove from heat, add remaining broth, and stir in Walnut Mayonnaise. Add onion, salt, and pepper. Chill for up to one hour—just until mixture starts to set. Fold in celery and pour into a 6-cup ring mold. Chill for 4–5 hours (or overnight).

Prepare chicken salad by mixing chicken, Walnut Mayonnaise, and celery. Arrange lettuce on round platter. When gelatin mold is chilled firm, unmold on lettuce bed. Fill center of ring with chicken salad. Arrange olives around outside of curried ring. Serve with crackers. *Serves 4–6.*

Chicken Broth

1½ quarts water
1 bay leaf
1 large onion, chopped
1 carrot, chopped
1½ pounds chicken breast

Pour water into a stockpot and add bay leaf, onion, and carrot. Bring to a boil. Add chicken (remove skins if too fatty) and reduce heat to low. Simmer for one hour. Remove chicken. Strain broth and store in jar in refrigerator. Bone chicken and use in chicken salad recipes. *Makes 5 cups.*

Note: You might be able to find canned yeast-free broth at the supermarket but remember that the general term "seasonings" can include yeast.

CHICKEN SALAD PLATTER

1 can Swanson's Chunk Chicken or ¾ cup cubed leftover cooked chicken
½ cup chopped red pepper
¼ cup Avocado Mayonnaise (see p. 56)
Boston lettuce
tomato slices (for sandwiches) or chunks (for plated salad)
celery sticks
black olives packed in water
rice cakes

Drain chicken and place in a mixing bowl with red pepper. Add Avocado Mayonnaise to taste. Arrange Boston lettuce and tomatoes on each plate and spoon chicken salad onto beds of lettuce. Garnish with celery sticks and olives. Serve with rice cakes. *For sandwiches,* spread chicken salad on rice cakes or 100% Plus Rye Bread (see p. 55). Top with lettuce leaf and tomato slice. Spread Avocado Mayonnaise on second rice cake or slice of bread and place on top. Sandwich or platter can be packed in container for lunch at work or on the go. *Serves 4.*

FISH CHOWDER

    1 onion, chopped
    3 celery stalks, chopped
    1 tablespoon olive oil
    ½ teaspoon salt
    1 cup rolled oats
    6 cups water
    ¼ teaspoon white pepper
    ½ teaspoon thyme
    ½ teaspoon basil
    1 bay leaf
    1 pound whitefish, cubed
       salt to taste (optional)

Sauté onion and celery in oil, adding the salt as mixture cooks. Stir in oats, water, herbs, and seasonings. Cook, covered, for 15 minutes. Blend one half in blender for creamy texture and return to pan. Add fish. Cook 10 minutes more. Season with salt to taste, if needed. Serve with crackers (see p. 55) and Grated Carrot Salad (see p. 93). *Serves 7–8.*

FRUIT SOUP AND GREEN GODDESS FRUIT SALAD

Fruit Soup
    3 cups pineapple juice
    1 banana
    1 chopped apple
    ¼ teaspoon ground cinnamon
    ¼ cup chopped fresh mint

Place all ingredients except mint in blender and blend well. Chill, covered, until ready to serve. Place in bowls and garnish with fresh mint. *Serves 4.*

Green Goddess Fruit Salad

    4 peaches, sliced
    1 honeydew melon, cubed
    2 apples, diced
    2 bananas, sliced
   ½ cup blueberries, whole strawberries, or raspberries
   ½ cup chopped walnuts
      Avocado Dressing (see p. 58)
      leafy lettuce

Combine fruit and nuts in a large bowl. Add Avocado Dressing and mix well. Arrange lettuce on plates or in portable plastic containers and spoon salad onto lettuce beds. *Serves 4.*

HAMBURGER WITH TOSSED SALAD*

    1 pound chopped beef
      Avocado Mayonnaise (see p. 56)
      100% Plus Rye Bread or rice cakes (see p. 55)

Form 4 hamburger patties and broil. Spread Avocado Mayonnaise on bread slices and place cooked hamburgers between two slices. *Serves 4.*

NOT DOGS

A word about the *Hot Dog That Is Not:* "Not Dogs" are soybean-derived hot dogs which are quite tasty. They are also a good source of protein. Produced by the Soyboy Corp., they can be bought or ordered at a health food store. You can cook and eat them hot, or cold the next day. Children love them cut into pieces and served on toothpicks. Dip in Homemade Mustard (see p. 58). Serve with rice cakes, Wasa Lite Rye Crackers, or 100% Plus Rye Bread (see p. 55) and raw vegetable sticks.

*For Tossed Salad, see pp. 94–95.

QUICK LUNCHES

Almond butter, cashew butter, hazelnut butter, and tahini are all sources of protein that stick to your ribs and are tasty on rice cakes or other crackers or breads listed on p. 55. This is great for that quick lunch when you're running late. You can buy all of these items at a health food store.

RICE BALLS

olive oil
leftover brown rice (best if sticky)
tofu, cubed
almonds
toasted sesame seeds

Oil your hands with olive oil. Take a small handful of leftover brown rice and form into a ball. Push a small cube of tofu or a couple of almonds in the middle and smooth back into a ball. Roll ball in toasted sesame seeds. Rice Balls are great for travel: no muss, no fuss. Serve with raw vegetable sticks or a salad.

SHRIMP SALAD WITH CREAM OF BROCCOLI SOUP

1   can tiny shrimp (see Appendix A)
½   cup chopped celery
½   cup chopped sweet red peppers
¼   cup Avocado Mayonnaise (see p. 56)
    ruby-leaf lettuce
1   zucchini, sliced
2   teaspoons chopped parsley

Drain shrimp and place in a bowl with celery, peppers, and mayonnaise. Mix well. Arrange ruby-leaf lettuce on individual plates. Make a ring of zucchini slices on top of lettuce bed. Spoon shrimp salad into center of ring. Garnish with chopped parsley. *Serves 2.*

Cream of Broccoli Soup
- 1½ cups chopped broccoli
- 2½ cups water
- ½ cup raw almonds or cashews
- 1 clove garlic
- ½ teaspoon salt
- 1 teaspoon fresh dill
- rice cakes

Cook broccoli in water, but do not overcook. Remove broccoli, reserving cooking water. Place almonds or cashews in a dry blender. Blend at high speed until very finely chopped. Reduce speed and slowly add the cooking water. Blend well. Add 1 cup of the cooked broccoli and the garlic, salt, and dill. Blend well. Stir in remaining ½ cup chopped broccoli. Serve immediately with rice cakes. May be reheated if necessary. *Serves 2.*

TOFU SALAD WITH QUICK CREAMED CARROT SOUP

- 1 package tofu, drained and mashed
  (tofu usually comes in 1 lb. blocks, packaged or in bulk)
- ½ can black olives, finely chopped
- ½ cup finely chopped celery
- ½ cup finely chopped red peppers
- ¼ cup toasted sesame seeds (see p. 59)
- 1–2 cloves garlic, minced
- ½ teaspoon salt
- ½ teaspoon curry powder
- 1 cup Walnut Mayonnaise (see p. 57)
- romaine lettuce
- 100% Plus Rye Bread, crackers, or rice cakes (see p. 55)

In a large bowl combine all ingredients except lettuce and bread. Mix well. Prepare a bed of lettuce and spoon tofu salad into center. Serve with bread or crackers on the side or spread tofu salad on bread or crackers and top with a lettuce leaf. *Serves 4.*

Quick Creamed Carrot Soup
>   5 cups water or chicken broth (see p. 67)
>   2½ cups grated carrots
>   ½ cup chopped onions
>   1 teaspoon powdered rosemary
>   1 teaspoon salt
>   1 cup raw almonds or cashews

Bring water or chicken broth to a boil. Add carrots, onions, rosemary, and salt. Reduce heat and simmer 5 minutes. Meanwhile, blend almonds or cashews in a dry blender at high speed. When carrot mixture is ready (the carrots will be soft), add to blender and blend at high speed. Serve immediately. *Serves 4.*

TUNA SALAD BOWL

>   1 can water-packed tuna or leftover cooked fish
>   ¾ cup finely chopped celery
>   ½ cup Walnut Mayonnaise (see p. 57)
>   romaine lettuce
>   sliced tomato
>   100% Plus Rye Bread or rice cakes (see p. 55)
>   carrot sticks

Drain tuna or leftover fish. Place in a bowl and flake using a fork. Add celery and mayonnaise to taste. Arrange romaine lettuce leaves and tomato slices on plates or in round container for portable lunch. Spoon tuna salad onto lettuce. Serve with bread or rice cakes and carrot sticks.

Variation: Tuna salad may be spread on bread or rice cakes and topped with lettuce and tomato for an open-face sandwich. *Serves 4.*

VEGGIE BURGERS

Veggie Burgers by the MudPie Co. are available in the freezer section of your health food store. Follow package directions. Serve with Homemade Mustard (see p. 58), rice cakes, and raw vegetables.

Dinner Recipes

In this section, we include dinner recipes for meat, fish, and poultry entrees, vegetarian entrees, side dishes, and salads. Following the recipes we give some menu ideas that will help you combine these dishes into tasty and well-balanced meals.

Meat, Fish, and Poultry Dinner Entrees for the Simplification Phase

- Marinated Stuffed Lamb Chops
- Liver and Onions with Béchamel Sauce
- Spanish Chicken
- Tangy Bluefish
- Stuffed Flounder
- Curried Fried Fish
- Cod Pie
- Poached Salmon
- Broiled Whitefish

The following recipes emphasize a healthy combination of fish and poultry. This does not mean you may not eat red meat (baked, broiled, or boiled). The message from research is clear, however, that eating less red meat and more fish and poultry leads to better overall health.

MARINATED STUFFED LAMB CHOPS

    4 very thick lamb chops (double)

Marinade:
    ¾ cup pineapple juice
    ¼ cup olive oil
    2 cloves garlic, minced
    1 teaspoon salt
    6 peppercorns (or ¼ teaspoon ground pepper)
    1 teaspoon oregano

Stuffing:
  ½ cup finely chopped fresh parsley
  2 tablespoons minced fresh onion
  ½ teaspoon powdered oregano
  ¼ teaspoon powdered rosemary
  2 tablespoons olive oil

Garnish:
  2 tablespoons chopped parsley

Place lamb chops in large, shallow baking dish. Slit the chops along the edge away from the bone to form a pocket (somewhat like pocket bread). Mix together all ingredients for marinade and marinate lamb for several hours or overnight in refrigerator (covered). Remove lamb from marinade. Lightly sauté parsley, onion, oregano, and rosemary in olive oil. Stuff chops with stuffing and seal openings with toothpicks. Broil on a rack two inches from heat. Brown on both sides (approximately 10 minutes per side). Serve garnished with fresh chopped parsley. *Serves 4.*

LIVER AND ONIONS WITH BÉCHAMEL SAUCE
Béchamel sauce:
  ¼ cup olive oil
  1 cup rye flour
  4 cups water
  ½ teaspoon salt
  ⅛ teaspoon pepper

Liver and onions:
  2 tablespoons olive oil
  2 onions, sliced in rings
  1½ pounds calf's liver (4 slices)

Step one: Begin by making béchamel sauce. Heat a skillet over medium heat (cast-iron skillets work best). Add the olive oil and flour. Stir and cook until flour is roasted and aromatic. Remove from skillet to a bowl. Cool. Mix water, salt, and pepper into cooled mixture with a whisk.

Step two: Using the same skillet, sauté onion rings lightly in olive oil. Remove onions from pan, add more oil if necessary, and quickly brown both sides of each piece of liver. Cover with béchamel sauce and place fried onion rings on top. Bring to boil, lower heat, cover skillet, and cook over low heat for 30 minutes, stirring occasionally. *Serves 4.*

SPANISH CHICKEN

        1 teaspoon salt
     1/2 teaspoon pepper
     1/8 teaspoon paprika
        2 pounds chicken pieces
     1/4 cup olive oil
        1 clove garlic, minced
        1 medium onion, chopped
     3/4 cup chopped green pepper
        2 cups water
    3 1/2 cups canned whole tomatoes
     1/2 teaspoon ground cumin
     1/8 teaspoon saffron
        1 bay leaf
     1/4 teaspoon salt
    1 1/2 cups raw brown rice

Preheat oven to 350°F. Mix salt, pepper, and paprika in a bowl. Roll chicken in mixture to coat. In skillet, quickly brown chicken pieces in olive oil. Remove and arrange chicken in a deep baking dish.

Using the same skillet, sauté garlic, onion, and green pepper until onion is transparent. Add water, tomatoes and their liquid, cumin, saffron, bay leaf, and salt. Bring to a boil, add rice, and pour over chicken. Cover. Bake 45 minutes. *Serves 4.*

TANGY BLUEFISH

    1 1/2 pounds bluefish, cod, or haddock fillets
        3 tablespoons olive oil
        1 teaspoon powdered mustard or powdered horseradish
     1/4 teaspoon garlic powder
           water
        1 cup finely chopped onion
     1/2 small can water-packed black pitted olives, sliced
     1/4 teaspoon salt or to taste

Preheat oven to 350°F. Rinse fish and place skin side down in a baking dish oiled with 1 tablespoon olive oil. Pat fish dry with paper towel. Mix mustard or horseradish and garlic powder with just enough water to make a paste. Top the fillets with a thin coat of this paste. Arrange chopped onion over the mustard paste and then the sliced olives on top of onions. Sprinkle with 2 tablespoons olive oil and salt. Bake 30–40 minutes, until fish flakes when pierced with fork. *Serves 4.*

STUFFED FLOUNDER/CHICKEN BREAST

> 1 tablespoon olive oil
> 1½ pounds flounder fillets

Stuffing:

> 1 clove garlic, minced
> 1 medium onion, chopped finely
> 1 tablespoon olive oil
> 2 cups cooked brown rice
> 2 teaspoons dried parsley
> 1 teaspoon basil
> ¼ cup rye flour
> ¾ cup boiling water

Topping:

> 2 tablespoons olive oil
> 2 tablespoons sesame seeds

Preheat oven to 350°F. Oil a baking dish with 1 tablespoon olive oil. Rinse flounder fillets in water and lay each fillet flat upon a work surface such as a tray or cutting board.

To prepare stuffing: In a skillet, sauté garlic and onion in olive oil over medium heat until onions are transparent. Add cooked rice, parsley, and basil. Mix well and cook 5 minutes over medium heat. In bowl, beat together the flour and boiling water. Pour into rice mixture in skillet, mixing well. Cook over low heat until mixture thickens (approximately 5–10 minutes).

Spoon 2 to 4 tablespoons stuffing (depending on size of the fillets) onto each fillet. Stuffing should be placed in a strip across the width and almost to one end of the fillet. Roll short end of fillet up and over the stuffing and continue rolling so that the stuffing is in the middle of the roll. Use toothpicks, if necessary, to hold in place.

Place rolled-up stuffed fillets in the baking dish with the overlapping end of each fillet on the bottom. Brush tops with olive oil. Sprinkle with sesame seeds. Bake 25 minutes. *Serves 4.*

Variation: This recipe may be used to make stuffed chicken breasts. Substitute boned chicken breasts for the flounder. If breasts are thick, pound thin. Lightly brown both sides of chicken in a skillet with olive oil over medium heat before stuffing. Baste with olive oil. Bake at 350°F , covered, for 20 minutes, then uncovered for 10 minutes. Baste with olive oil during cooking as needed.

CURRIED FRIED FISH

        2 tablespoons olive oil
    1½ pounds fish fillets
    1½ cups rye or oat flour
        1 teaspoon salt
      ½ teaspoon pepper
        1 teaspoon curry powder

Heat a cast-iron skillet or frying pan over medium heat. Add oil. Rinse fish fillets in water. Mix flour, salt, pepper, and curry powder in a shallow dish. Dip each fillet in flour mixture and fry both sides (approximately 5–10 minutes per side) in oil. Fish is done when it flakes easily with a fork. *Serves 4.*

COD PIE

Pie crust:
        3 cups rye flour
      ½ teaspoon salt
      ½ cup olive oil or soft soy margarine
      ¾ cup cold water
            waxed paper (for rolling crust)

Filling:

    1 pound cod or pollock fillets
    ¼ cup water
    ¼ teaspoon salt
    1 bay leaf
    1 chopped onion
    1 clove garlic, minced
    3 tablespoons chopped celery
    ¼ cup olive oil
    ¼ cup rye flour
    ½ cup whole walnuts
 1¾ cups water
    ½ teaspoon dry mustard
    ¼ cup chopped walnuts
    1 tablespoon chopped red pepper

Step one: Preheat oven to 400°F. Make crust: Combine flour and salt in a large bowl. Add the oil or soy margarine and stir it into the flour with a fork until flour has a pebbly consistency. Add enough water to moisten dough so that it forms a large ball. Divide ball in half and reserve one portion for later. Roll out crust between two pieces of waxed paper that have been dusted with rye flour (wet surface of countertop before putting down waxed paper to avoid slippage when rolling dough). Peel off top piece of waxed paper and place dough circle upside down in a nine-inch pie dish. Remove second piece of waxed paper. Prick bottom of crust. Bake for 5 minutes.

Step two: While pie crust is baking, place the fish, water, salt, and bayleaf in a large skillet. Cover. Bring to a boil, reduce the heat, and simmer for 5 minutes. Remove fish; drain and flake.

Over medium heat sauté onion, garlic, and celery in olive oil until soft. Stir in the flour and cook for 1 minute over low heat. In a blender, chop ½ cup walnuts very fine by turning the blender on and off. With blender on, slowly add water and dry mustard and blend at high speed until creamy.

Slowly add this "walnut milk" to sautéed onions and flour mixture, stirring constantly over low heat until mixture thickens and bubbles—approximately 3–5 minutes. Remove from heat. Add ¼ cup chopped walnuts, red pepper, and flaked fish. Mix well and pour into crust.

Using ball of dough set aside earlier, roll out top crust and place over filling. Crimp edges of both crusts together to seal. Cut steam vents in top crust for steam to escape. Bake 30 minutes, until top crust is golden brown. Remove from oven and let cool 10–15 minutes before cutting. Cod pie slices can be taken to work or school the next day for lunch! *Serves 6.*

POACHED SALMON

     water
     pinch of salt
1½ pounds salmon fillets

Sauce:
½ cup rolled oats
¼ teaspoon salt
1 large onion, diced
2 cups water
1 tablespoon tahini

Garnish:
     chopped parsley

Bring a medium skillet full of water to a boil. Add pinch of salt. Place fresh fillets of salmon in water. Poach until done (approximately 10 minutes—salmon should be light pink). Remove. While salmon is poaching, mix sauce ingredients together in a saucepan and cook over medium heat for 15 minutes, then pour into blender and blend until smooth. Place salmon on serving dish and pour sauce over. Garnish with parsley. *Serves 4.*

BROILED WHITEFISH

1½ pounds whitefish fillets
2 tablespoons olive oil
¼ teaspoon salt
½ teaspoon basil

Brush whitefish fillets with a mixture of olive oil, salt, and basil. Place on piece of oiled foil and broil two inches from heat for approximately 6–10 minutes, or until done (flakes easily with a fork). *Serves 4.*

Vegetarian Dinner Entrees for the Simplification Phase

- Baked Stuffed Squash
- Potato-Leek Soup
- Mexican Beans with Enchilada Sauce
- Stir-Fried Vegetables and Tofu
- Light and Lovely Split Pea Soup
- Sunny Burgers with Tomato Sauce
- Vegetable Barley Soup
- Tofu with Sauce
- Indian Pulao with Indian Curried Vegetables
- Black Bean Soup

BAKED STUFFED SQUASH

    2 small or 1 large acorn squash
       water

Stuffing:

    1½ apples, chopped
    ½   cup chopped celery
    ¼   cup water
    1   teaspoon olive oil
    1½ cups cooked brown rice
    1–2 tablespoons honey
    1   teaspoon ground cinnamon
    ½   teaspoon ground nutmeg
    ¼   teaspoon salt
    ½   cup walnuts, coarsely chopped, or sunflower seeds

Preheat oven to 400°F. Cut squash in half, from tip to stem. Remove seeds. Place cut side down in baking pan with ½ inch water in bottom. Bake for 20 minutes. While squash is baking, cook apples and celery in saucepan with oil and water to prevent sticking until soft. Add remaining ingredients and mix. Remove squash from oven. Turn each piece over and stuff. Return to oven (stuffing side up). Bake until squash is tender—another 20–30 minutes. *Serves 4.*

POTATO-LEEK SOUP

    1 stalk celery, sliced
    1 large onion, chopped
    2 cloves garlic, minced
  2–3 leeks, sliced thinly
    4 tablespoons olive oil
    3 medium potatoes, cubed
  3–4 cups water
   ½ teaspoon salt
    1 teaspoon marjoram
   ½ pound tofu, cut into ½-inch cubes

Garnish:
  2–4 tablespoons minced fresh parsley

Sauté celery, onion, garlic, and leeks in oil until they are soft but still retain their color. Set aside. Boil potatoes in water with salt and marjoram until soft. Add sautéed celery mixture to potatoes. Boil for 5 minutes. Remove one quarter to one half of this mixture and place in blender. Add tofu and blend at medium speed until creamy. Return to pot over low heat. Adjust liquid and salt to taste. Garnish hot soup with parsley just before serving. *Serves 4.*

MEXICAN BEANS WITH ENCHILADA SAUCE
Mexican Beans:
    1 onion, chopped
  2–3 cloves garlic, minced
    4 tablespoons olive oil
    2 tablespoons chili powder
   ½ teaspoon cumin
   ½ teaspoon basil
   ½ teaspoon salt
    4 cups well-cooked pinto or kidney beans (see Cooking Legumes, page 53); reserve stock
       Enchilada Sauce (recipe follows)

Sauté onion and garlic in olive oil. Add spices, salt, beans, and enough water or stock to keep moist. Mash beans with potato masher or pastry blender. Add liquid, if needed, until beans are consistency of lumpy mashed potatoes. Adjust seasonings to taste. Top with Enchilada Sauce. *Serves 4–6.*

Enchilada Sauce

        2   tablespoons olive oil
        2   tablespoons rye flour
        3   cups bean stock or water
        1   8-ounce can tomato sauce
      ½   teaspoon salt
    ¾–1   teaspoon cumin
        1   tablespoon chili powder
      ½   teaspoon garlic powder

Mix oil and flour in saucepan over medium heat. Gradually add bean stock or water, mixing thoroughly. Add remaining ingredients. Bring to boil, stirring constantly, until thickened to consistency of thin gravy. Adjust seasoning to taste. Spoon over Mexican Beans.

Other serving suggestions:

1. *Easy Serve.* Place a mound of beans and a mound of rice on each plate. Pour hot enchilada sauce over both. Top with shredded lettuce, chopped fresh tomatoes, chopped onion, and chopped green pepper.

2. *Quick Enchilada.* Place a spoonful of beans on a cooked Rye Flour Tortilla (see p. 91). Roll tortilla around beans. Place on dinner plate with a mound of rice and pour sauce over both. Top tortilla with shredded lettuce and chopped fresh tomatoes, onion, and green pepper.

3. *Baked Enchiladas.* Roll beans in tortillas as above. Place in baking pan and cover with sauce. Cover and bake in oven until bubbly. Serve with rice, shredded lettuce, and chopped fresh tomatoes, onion, and green pepper.

STIR-FRIED VEGETABLES AND TOFU

¼	cup sesame or olive oil
½–1	pound tofu, cubed
1	large onion, thinly sliced
1	stalk celery, thinly sliced at an angle
1	large carrot cut in matchstick slices
2	cups thinly sliced Chinese or regular cabbage
1	cup minced fresh parsley
1	cup canned or fresh soybean sprouts, drained
1	cup toasted chopped almonds
1	tablespoon grated fresh ginger or ½ teaspoon ginger powder
½	teaspoon salt (or to taste)

Heat oil in pan. Lightly brown tofu and set aside. Sauté vegetables in the following order (cooking 1–2 minutes between each addition): onion, celery, carrot, cabbage. Add parsley, soybean sprouts, almonds, ginger, salt, and tofu. Stir gently, cooking for 1 minute. Toss lightly and serve over brown rice. *Serves 4–6.*

Note: The secret of stir-frying is to stir as little as possible—just lightly coat each ingredient with oil, add next ingredient, and continue in the same way.

LIGHT AND LOVELY SPLIT PEA SOUP

3	stalks celery, chopped
1	small carrot, chopped
1	medium onion, chopped
2	cloves garlic, minced, or ½ teaspoon garlic powder
2	tablespoons olive oil
6	cups water
1	cup dry green or yellow split peas
1	bay leaf
6	cups sliced or cubed zucchini
½	teaspoon basil
1½	teaspoon salt (or to taste)
4	tablespoons minced fresh parsley

Sauté celery, carrot, onion, and garlic in oil until tender. In another pot, bring water to boil. Add peas, bay leaf, and sautéed celery–carrot mixture. Cover and simmer until peas are tender and beginning to crumble, about 45 minutes. While peas are cooking, prepare zucchini. When peas are tender, add zucchini, basil, and salt. Continue cooking until zucchini become translucent, about 10 minutes. Adjust salt and water. Remove bay leaf. Serve as is with parsley on top, or blend for a smooth, creamy soup. (Even pea soup critics like this version.) *Serves 6–8.*

SUNNY BURGERS WITH TOMATO SAUCE

     2 cups grated carrots
     1 medium onion, finely chopped
    ½ cup rolled oats or ½ cup rye flour
    ¾ cup sunflower seeds, ground in blender
    ¾ cup cooked chick peas, mashed or puréed in blender
    ½ teaspoon basil
     2 tablespoons olive oil
     1 teaspoon salt
        water or bean stock (optional)
        sesame seeds
        olive oil for frying
        Tomato Sauce (recipe follows)

In bowl, mix all ingredients except water or bean stock, sesame seeds, and oil for frying. Add water or bean stock if necessary so that mixture can be formed into patties. Form patties. Sprinkle with sesame seeds on both sides. Fry in oil until golden brown. Serve with Tomato Sauce. *Serves 4–6.*

Tomato Sauce

     4 cups canned chopped tomatoes, with juice
     1 small carrot, grated
     1 green pepper, chopped finely
     1 medium onion, chopped finely

    1 small can tomato paste
  ¼ cup olive oil
    3 cloves garlic, minced
  ½ teaspoon basil
  ½ teaspoon oregano
  ½ teaspoon marjoram
  ½ teaspoon salt

Mix all ingredients in large saucepan. Cover. Bring to boil and simmer 45 minutes. Serve hot over Sunny Burgers. This sauce can also be stored in a jar in the refrigerator and used as ketchup with other dishes. *Makes 1 quart.*

VEGETABLE BARLEY SOUP

    1 leek or medium onion, chopped
    2 cloves garlic, minced
    3 tablespoons olive oil
    8 cups water
    1 cup raw barley
    2 cups sliced carrots
    1 cup sliced celery
    2 cups chopped tomatoes (optional)
  ½ teaspoon tarragon
  ½ teaspoon marjoram
  ½ teaspoon thyme
    1 bay leaf
    2 teaspoons salt
    2 cups fresh or frozen peas
    2 cups chopped Swiss chard, kale, or spinach
    2 tablespoons chopped fresh parsley

Sauté leek and garlic in oil until tender. Add water. Bring to boil. Add barley and simmer, covered, for 1 hour. Add carrots, celery, tomatoes (if desired), and seasonings. Simmer 30–45 minutes longer. Ten minutes before serving, add peas. Cook 5 minutes. Add chard, kale, or spinach and parsley. Cook another few minutes. Adjust salt to taste. Serve hot. *Serves 8.*

TOFU WITH SAUCE

        2 onions, thinly sliced
        2 carrots, thinly sliced
        2 tablespoons olive oil
     ½ pound tofu, diced
        1 tablespoon arrowroot
     ½ cup water

Sauté onions and carrots in olive oil for 5 minutes. Add tofu to mixture and stir-fry. Meanwhile, mix arrowroot and water in a small cup until smooth. Add to stir-fry mixture and stir until sauce becomes thick and clear. *Serves 2.*

INDIAN PULAO WITH
INDIAN CURRIED VEGETABLES

     ⅓ cup olive oil
     1½ cups basmati rice*
        4 cups water
     4½ tablespoons olive oil
     ¾ teaspoon mustard seeds
     1½ teaspoon turmeric
     1½ cups green peas
     ¾ cup chopped green pepper
        18 cashews, chopped
     1½ teaspoons salt
     2¼ teaspoons curry powder
     ½ teaspoon honey
        Indian Curried Vegetables (recipe follows)

In a saucepan, heat oil and add rice. Sauté rice over low heat for 3 minutes or until it turns a pale gold color. Add water, cover, and cook until tender—about 30–45 minutes. Set cooked rice aside to cool. In another pan, heat oil; add mustard seeds. When seeds begin to pop, add turmeric, peas, and green pepper. Cook for 3–4 minutes. Add cashews, mixing well. Stir in cooked rice, salt, curry powder, and honey. Mix well. Serve with Indian Curried Vegetables. *Serves 4.*

*You can purchase basmati rice at a health food store or use plain, long-grain brown rice.

INDIAN CURRIED VEGETABLES

    1 large onion, chopped
    2 cloves garlic, minced
    2 tablespoons olive oil
    1 tablespoon curry powder
    ¼ teaspoon ground cinnamon
    1 teaspoon salt
    1 cup water
    2 large carrots, sliced
    1 large potato, boiled and cubed
    1 large zucchini, sliced
    1 16-ounce can whole tomatoes, chopped

Sauté onion and garlic in oil. Stir in curry, cinnamon, salt, and water. Bring to a boil and add carrots, potato, and zucchini. Cover and simmer for 15 minutes. Add tomatoes. Simmer for 10 minutes. Serve hot. *Serves 4.*

BLACK BEAN SOUP

    1 cup cooked black beans (see Cooking Legumes, page 53)
    3 cups water
    1 medium onion, finely diced
    1 stalk celery, finely diced
    1 large carrot, finely diced
    1 tablespoon olive or sesame oil
    1 teaspoon salt
    ½ teaspoon garlic powder or 1 garlic clove, crushed
    ½ teaspoon basil
    ½ cup chopped fresh parsley
    1 bay leaf

Garnish:
        chopped fresh parsley

Place beans and water in a pot and bring to a boil. Sauté onion, celery, and carrot in oil and salt until tender. Stir this mixture into beans, adding garlic, basil, parsley, and bay leaf. Simmer for 15 minutes. Garnish with parsley. *Serves 4.*

Side Dishes for the Simplification Phase

- Autumn Casserole
- Brown Rice Plus
- Butternut Bisque
- Cauliflower with Cashew Gravy
- Cranberry Sauce
- French Fries
- Gingered Carrots
- Italian Greens
- Rye Flour Tortillas
- Sesame Broccoli Especiale
- Sesame Greens
- Springtime Rice Salad

AUTUMN CASSEROLE

>   2 onions, sliced
>   2 tablespoons olive oil
>   2 yams (or equivalent amounts of an orange root vegetable:
>   1 rutabaga, 4 carrots, or 2 sweet potatoes), peeled and
>   sliced thinly
>   2 medium parsnips, 1 large potato, or 2 turnips, sliced thinly
>   1–2 apples, sliced thinly
>   ½ medium red cabbage, sliced thinly
>   water or apple juice
>   chopped almonds, filberts, walnuts, or pumpkin seeds

Preheat oven to 400°F. Sauté onions in olive oil until translucent.
Choose two of your favorite root vegetables from those listed above.
Layer them with sautéed onions, apples, and cabbage in a shallow
oiled baking dish. Add water or apple juice to cover bottom of dish.
Cover and bake until vegetables are very soft, approximately 50–
60 minutes. When vegetables are done (vegetables may be steamed
before baking to reduce baking time in oven), remove cover and
sprinkle with chopped nuts or seeds. Bake, uncovered, until nuts
or seeds are golden brown. Serve hot. *Serves 6.*

BROWN RICE PLUS

        2 cups brown rice
        3 cups water
        1 tablespoon sesame oil
        1 medium onion, finely chopped
        1 large carrot, grated
        1 large stalk celery, chopped
    2–3 cloves garlic, minced
        3 scallions, sliced (including tops)

Preheat oven to 375°F. Mix together ingredients in order given. Pour into oiled casserole dish. Cover and bake for 60 minutes. *Serves 4.*

BUTTERNUT BISQUE

        1 medium butternut squash, cooked
        2 tablespoons tahini (more if desired)
        1 small onion, chopped
        1 clove garlic, minced or crushed
        1 leek, thinly sliced
      ½ stalk celery, chopped
        1 tablespoon olive oil

Blend squash well in blender until smooth. Add tahini and blend until creamy. Sauté onions, garlic, leek, and celery in oil. Add to soup and warm over gentle heat. Do not boil. *Serves 4.*

CAULIFLOWER WITH CASHEW GRAVY

        1 medium cauliflower, broken into flowerettes and steamed

Cashew gravy:
      ½ cup ground, raw cashews
        1 small onion, chopped
        2 tablespoons olive oil
        4 tablespoons rye or rice flour
        2 cups water
        1 teaspoon salt (or to taste)
        2 tablespoons finely chopped scallions or chives (optional)

Prepare gravy while cauliflower steams: Grind dry cashews in blender and set aside. Sauté onion in oil over medium heat until translucent. Add flour and ground cashews. Cook several minutes, stirring constantly. Add water slowly, stirring constantly. Continue cooking and stirring until gravy thickens. Blend in blender until smooth. Reheat, if needed, and add salt and scallions or chives, if desired. Pour over steamed cauliflower. *Serves 4.*

CRANBERRY SAUCE

    1 bag fresh or frozen cranberries
    1 cup water
¼–½ cup maple syrup or honey
   ½ cup chopped walnuts
    1 cup halved and seeded grapes (preferably red)

Steam cranberries 5–10 minutes in water, until berries burst. Remove from heat and add maple syrup or honey and walnuts. Chill. Stir in grapes before serving. *Serves 6.*

FRENCH FRIES

    1 large potato per person
       olive oil
       salt

Preheat oven to 450°F. Scrub potatoes. Slice into strips, leaving skins on. Use hands to toss potatoes in large bowl with enough oil to coat each piece. Spread potatoes on oiled baking sheet in single layer and sprinkle lightly with salt. Bake until tender—about 30 to 40 minutes. Turn fries. Place under broiler to brown for a minute or two, then turn again to brown other side. Serve plain or with Tomato Sauce (see p. 84).

GINGERED CARROTS

    4 cups carrots, thinly sliced
    2 tablespoons sesame oil
    2 teaspoons rye or rice flour

¼ cup water
¼ teaspoon grated fresh ginger root or pinch ginger powder
   (to taste)
½ teaspoon salt
 2 tablespoons almond slivers (optional)

Sauté carrots in oil for 5 minutes. Add flour and mix thoroughly. Slowly add water and ginger. Cover and simmer until tender. Add salt and garnish with almond slivers. *Serves 4–6.*

ITALIAN GREENS

 1 large bunch of greens (kale, collards, cabbage, spinach, or
   other, or a mixture)
 1 clove garlic, diced or pressed
 2 tablespoons olive oil
¼ teaspoon salt
¼ cup water

Chop greens. Place in a pot. Place garlic on top of greens. Sprinkle with oil and salt. Pour water down side of pot. Cover and bring to a boil, simmer 5 minutes, then stir. Continue to cook until greens are tender, but still retain green color. This can be as short as three minutes. Do not overcook! *Serves 4.*

RYE FLOUR TORTILLAS

 2 cups rye flour
½ cup plus 2 tablespoons water
¼–½ teaspoon salt
¼ cup olive oil

Mix all ingredients in large bowl, then knead on floured board 5 minutes. Keep board dusted with flour to keep dough from sticking. Shape into six-inch log-shaped roll. Cut into eight equal pieces. Flatten and roll into six-inch tortillas. Stack on plate, cover with plastic wrap, and store in refrigerator until ready to use. Cook one by one on both sides in lightly oiled skillet until lightly browned and bubbles appear. Stack and serve hot. *Makes eight six-inch tortillas.*

SESAME BROCCOLI ESPECIALE

2–3 bunches broccoli
 ½ teaspoon marjoram
1–2 tablespoons toasted sesame seeds (see p. 59)
 1 small carrot, grated (optional)

Cut tops of broccoli into large flowerettes. Slice stalks very thinly. Toss together with marjoram. Steam until tender. Sprinkle with sesame seeds and toss lightly. Garnish with grated carrot. *Serves 4–6.*

SESAME GREENS

 ½ small cabbage (savoy or green), finely chopped
 1 small bunch of your favorite green leafy vegetable (kale, collards, mustard greens, broccoli rabe, broccoli, beet greens, or carrot tops)
 1 small carrot
 1 cup toasted sesame seeds (see p. 59)
 ¼–½ teaspoon salt
 ⅛–¼ cup water

Place cabbage in medium-size pot. Rinse and chop greens; place on top of cabbage. Cut carrot into matchstick slices and place on top of greens. In blender, blend sesame seeds and salt into a powder. Pour on top of vegetables. Add water, cover and bring to a boil. Lower heat and simmer for 15 minutes, stirring after 5 minutes and again at end of 15 minutes. Turn into serving dish. *Serves 4.*

SPRINGTIME RICE SALAD

 3 scallions, finely diced
 2 stalks celery, finely chopped
 1 large carrot, grated
 7 radishes, sliced thinly
 2 pickling cucumbers or 1 cucumber, sliced thinly
 1 small bunch parsley, minced
 2 cups cooked brown rice
 ¾ cup salad dressing of choice (see pp. 58–59)

Garnish:
Carrot flowerettes or chopped watercress

Combine all ingredients in mixing bowl. Toss gently but thoroughly. Transfer into serving bowl. Garnish with carrot flowers or watercress. *Serves 6.*

Variations: You may add any or all of the following: ½ cup cooked peas; ½ cup cooked string beans, chopped; 1 small bunch watercress, chopped; or use barley instead of rice.

Salads for the Simplification Phase

- Carrot-Pineapple Salad
- Grated Carrot Salad
- Three-Bean Salad
- Tomato-Cucumber Salad
- Tossed Salad

CARROT-PINEAPPLE SALAD

4–6 large carrots, grated
1 tablespoon olive oil
1 small can crushed pineapple in its own juice, drained

Mix all ingredients together in bowl. *Serves 4.*

GRATED CARROT SALAD

4 carrots, grated
¼ cup salad dressing of choice (see pp. 58–59)

Garnish:
chopped parsley

Mix ingredients together and serve as is or chill if desired. Garnish with parsley. *Serves 2–4.*

THREE-BEAN SALAD

  1   cup cooked garbanzo beans (see Cooking Legumes, p. 53)
  1   cup cooked kidney beans (see Cooking Legumes, p. 53)
  1   cup lightly steamed green string beans, cut in one-inch pieces
  1   cup lightly steamed yellow string beans, cut in one-inch pieces
  2+ tablespoons minced onion
  1   clove garlic, minced (optional)
  3   tablespoons chopped fresh parsley
  2   cups chopped ripe tomatoes, with juice
  1   teaspoon basil
  ½   teaspoon salt
  1   tablespoon olive oil

Mix all ingredients together; chill. *Serves 6.*

TOMATO-CUCUMBER SALAD

  1   cucumber
  2   cups chopped fresh tomatoes
  ½   cup chopped celery
  2   tablespoons minced onion
  1   green pepper, chopped
  1   teaspoon basil
  ¼   teaspoon salt
      ground pepper to taste
  1   clove garlic, finely minced, or ½ teaspoon garlic powder (optional)
      salad dressing of choice (see pp. 58–59)

Peel cucumber. Cut lengthwise into quarters and slice. Prepare remaining vegetables. Mix all ingredients together. Chill. Serve with salad dressing. *Serves 4.*

TOSSED SALAD

  ½   head romaine lettuce, broken up
  1   tomato, cubed
  1   summer squash, sliced
  3   stalks celery, diced

    ½ cup sliced purple cabbage
    ½ cup grated carrot
    ¾ cup Avocado Mayonnaise (see p. 56)
    ⅓ cup water

Toss vegetables together. Blend Avocado Mayonnaise with water until smooth. Serve with tossed salad. *Serves 4.*

Dinner Menus

Here are some dinner menu suggestions to help you combine the recipes on the previous pages into nutritious and delicious meals. Use any of the desserts listed on pages 96–104 for a grand finish to your dinner.

1. Marinated Stuffed Lamb Chops (pp. 73–74) or Baked Stuffed
     Squash (pp. 80–81)
   Cauliflower with Cashew Gravy (pp. 89–90)
   Green beans or peas
   Cranberry Sauce (p. 90)
   Tossed Salad (pp. 94–95)

2. Liver and Onions with Béchamel Sauce (pp. 74–75) or Potato-
     Leek Soup (p. 81)
   Springtime Rice Salad (pp. 92–93)
   Italian Greens (p. 91)
   Steamed beets

3. Spanish Chicken (p. 75) or Mexican Beans with Enchilada Sauce
     (pp. 81–82)
   Brown rice
   Tomato-Cucumber Salad (p. 94)
   Rye Flour Tortillas (p. 91) or Wasa Lite Rye Crackers

4. Tangy Bluefish (pp. 75–76) or Stir-Fried Vegetables and Tofu
     (p. 83)
   Brown Rice Plus (p. 89)
   Baked sweet potatoes
   Tossed Salad (pp. 94–95)

5. Stuffed Flounder or Stuffed Chicken Breasts (pp. 76–77) or
     Light and Lovely Split Pea Soup (pp. 83–84)
   Brown Rice
   Gingered Carrots (pp. 90–91)
   Tossed Salad (pp. 94–95)

6. Curried Fried Fish (p. 77) or Sunny Burgers with Tomato Sauce
     (pp. 89–90)
   French Fries (p. 90)
   Sesame Broccoli Especiale (p. 92)
   Carrot-Pineapple Salad (p. 93)

7. Cod Pie (pp. 77–78) or Vegetable Barley Soup (p. 85)
   Steamed or sautéed zucchini
   Wasa Lite Rye Crackers
   Three-Bean Salad (p. 94)

Dessert Recipes for the Simplification Phase

- Accidental Mousse
- Almond Cookies
- Apple Crisp with Tofu Whipped Cream
- Baked Apples
- Banana Bread
- Banana Ice Cream
- Blueberry Kanten
- Cashew-Coconut Cookies
- Fresh Fruit Salad
- Hazelnut Cookies
- Homemade Applesauce
- Millet-Banana Bread
- Oatmeal-Rice Cookies
- Pumpkin Cream Pie
- Rice Dream Ice Cream or Sorbet
- Tahini Custard

ACCIDENTAL MOUSSE

1½ cups unsweetened applesauce (commercial or homemade;
      see p. 101)
  6 very ripe bananas, cut into two-inch pieces

2 tablespoons carob powder
¼ teaspoon alcohol-free vanilla extract (see pp. 59–60)

This delicious dessert is made from readily available unprocessed natural ingredients. No sugar or sweeteners are added.

Blend the applesauce and bananas in a food processor fitted with a steel blade or in a blender. Add the carob powder and vanilla extract. Continue to blend until the mixture is smooth and all of the bananas have been completely blended. Pour into individual dessert cups or a large bowl. Refrigerate for 30 minutes. (The pectin in the apples makes this very loose mixture set after about ½ hour.) *Serves 4.*

ALMOND COOKIES

olive oil
¼ cup sesame oil
½ cup maple syrup
½ cup almond butter
1 teaspoon alcohol-free vanilla extract (see pp. 59–60)
3 tablespoons water
1 cup oat flour
1 cup rice flour
½ cup toasted almonds, chopped
whole almonds

Preheat oven to 350°F. Grease cookie sheet with olive oil. Mix together all ingredients, except whole almonds, in order given. Drop batter by tablespoons onto cookie sheet. Top with one whole almond pressed down in the center of each cookie. Bake 12–15 minutes. *Makes 2 dozen.*

APPLE CRISP WITH TOFU WHIPPED CREAM

approximately 6 apples, cored and sliced thinly (skins on)
1 cup rolled oats
½ cup honey
1 teaspoon ground cinnamon
¼ cup soy oil or melted soy margarine
apple juice, cider, or water
Tofu Whipped Cream (recipe follows; optional)

Preheat oven to 375°F. Fill two-quart baking dish with sliced apples. Mix together oats, honey, cinnamon, and oil or margarine. Crumble over top of apples. Pour in enough apple juice, cider, or water to cover bottom of baking dish. Bake 30 minutes. Top each serving with Tofu Whipped Cream, if desired. *Serves 4–6.*

Tofu Whipped Cream
      2 cups tofu
    ½ cup soy oil
    ⅓ cup plus 2 tablespoons honey
  1¼ teaspoons alcohol-free vanilla extract (see pp. 59–60)
      4 tablespoons soy milk (see p. 57)

Blend all ingredients together in a blender until smooth. Pour into bowl, cover, and chill for one hour or overnight before serving. This is an excellent nondairy topping. *Makes approximately 3 cups.*

BAKED APPLES
      4 baking apples
          boiling water

Filling #1:
      4 teaspoons tahini
      4 teaspoons maple syrup
      2 teaspoons chopped walnuts
      1 teaspoon sesame seeds

Filling #2:
      4 teaspoons almond butter
      4 teaspoons honey or rice syrup
      2 teaspoons chopped almonds

Filling #3:
      4 teaspoons maple syrup
      2 teaspoons soy margarine

Preheat oven to 375°F. Core apples, leaving one-half inch at bottom. Place apples in shallow baking dish and stuff with filling of choice.

Fillings may be made by combining ingredients listed. Pour boiling water around apples to cover bottom of baking dish. Cover and bake for 40–50 minutes, or until apples are soft and bubbly. Serve hot or chilled. *Serves 4.*

BANANA BREAD

olive oil
1½ cups brown rice flour and/or oat flour
4 teaspoons corn-free baking powder (see p. 54)
pinch each salt and ground cinnamon, nutmeg, and cloves
4 ripe bananas, mashed
½ cup sunflower oil
¾ cup honey
4 egg equivalents (see p. 56)
1⅓ cups chopped walnuts

Preheat oven to 350°F. Grease a 9 × 3 × 5-inch bread pan. In bowl, mix ingredients in order given. Pour into prepared pan and bake until golden brown and toothpick comes out clean (approximately 50 minutes). *Makes 2 small loaves.*

BANANA ICE CREAM

4–6 very ripe bananas (well speckled)
apple juice or water

Freeze bananas (just put in freezer as they are). When frozen, pare off skins with knife. Chop into small pieces and place in blender or food processor. Begin at slow speed, adding just enough water or apple juice to allow bananas to blend easily. When entirely whipped, eat right away or put in container and return to freezer immediately. *Serves 4.*

Variation: You can make this recipe using 2–3 frozen bananas and an equal amount of fresh strawberries, raspberries, blueberries, or canned unsweetened crushed pineapple.

BLUEBERRY KANTEN

        1 pint fresh blueberries
     3½ cups water
       ½ cup maple syrup or honey
       ½ teaspoon salt
        2 packages plain gelatin or 5 tablespoons agar-agar flakes*

Garnish:
        1 kiwi fruit

Rinse blueberries and place in saucepan with water, maple syrup or honey, salt, and gelatin or agar-agar flakes. Mix well. Bring to a boil. Lower flame and simmer for 3 minutes. Pour into a wet mold. Chill until hardened (approximately 4 hours). Unmold and garnish with sliced kiwi. *Serves 4.*

*Agar-agar flakes can be purchased at a health food store. They are a sea-vegetable derivative.

CASHEW-COCONUT COOKIES

            olive oil
       ½ cup sesame oil
       ½ cup maple syrup
        4 tablespoons almond butter
       ½ cup water
        1 teaspoon alcohol-free vanilla extract (see pp. 59–60)
       ¾ cup dried flaked coconut
     3½ cups rolled oats
        1 cup rice flour
        1 teaspoon salt
        1 cup chopped cashews
            water, if needed

Preheat oven to 350°F. Grease cookie sheet with olive oil. Mix together wet ingredients, then stir in dry ingredients in order given. Add just enough water, if needed, to make a sticky dough. Drop by tablespoons onto cookie sheet. Bake 15–20 minutes, or until light brown. *Makes 3 dozen.*

FRESH FRUIT SALAD

Cut your favorite fruits (those on the "allowable" food list) into bite-size chunks and place in a bowl. A sauce can be made by blending part of the fruit salad in a blender until smooth.

HAZELNUT COOKIES

        olive oil
   ½ cup sesame oil
   ½ cup maple syrup
   2 teaspoons alcohol-free vanilla extract (see pp. 59–60; optional)
 1½ cups ground toasted hazelnuts or sesame seeds (see p. 59)
   1 cup oat flour
   1 cup rice flour
   ¼ teaspoon salt
        unsweetened raspberry jam*

Preheat oven to 350°F. Grease cookie sheets with olive oil. Stir sesame oil and maple syrup together. Add vanilla, if using. Grind nuts or seeds in dry blender. Stir nuts, flours, and salt into liquid mixture. Wet hands and roll dough into 1½-inch balls. Place two inches apart on cookie sheet. Flatten balls and make indentation in center. Fill with raspberry jam. Bake 15–20 minutes, or until light brown. *Makes about 2 dozen.*

*Available at health food stores.

HOMEMADE APPLESAUCE

        cooking apples, cored and quartered (with skin)
        water
        pinch of salt

Wash and cut apples, then place in saucepan. Add enough water to cover the bottom of the pot. Add pinch of salt, then bring to boil. Cover and simmer until apples are soft (approximately 20 minutes). Blend in blender. Store in a jar in refrigerator. A *great* substitute for maple syrup.

MILLET-BANANA BREAD

    olive oil
1 cup mashed bananas
1 egg equivalent (see p. 56)
¼ cup sesame oil
⅓ cup maple syrup
2 tablespoons tahini
1 cup millet flour or rice flour
1 teaspoon baking soda
½ cup chopped walnuts
½ teaspoon salt

Preheat oven to 350°F. Grease 9 × 3 × 5-inch bread pan with olive oil. Combine ingredients in order given. Pour into prepared pan. Bake until golden brown on top (approximately 45–50 minutes). *Makes 1 loaf.*

OATMEAL-RICE COOKIES

    olive oil
¾ cup sesame or sunflower oil
¾ cup honey
3 egg equivalents (see p. 56)
¼ cup water
1 teaspoon alcohol-free vanilla extract (see pp. 59–60)
3 cups rolled oats
½ cup oat flour
½ cup rice flour
1 teaspoon baking soda
½ teaspoon salt

Preheat oven to 350°F. Grease cookie sheet with olive oil. Mix together wet ingredients. In separate bowl, mix together dry ingredients. Stir in wet ingredients. Drop onto cookie sheet by heaping tablespoons in rows. Bake 12–15 minutes, or until golden brown. *Makes about 5 dozen.*

PUMPKIN CREAM PIE
Oat-nut crust (no flour):
- ½ cup ground almonds
- ½ cup ground walnuts
- 1 cup rolled oats
- ¼ teaspoon sea salt
- ¼ cup water
- ⅛ cup maple syrup
- 4 tablespoons sesame oil

Pie filling:
- 1½ cups cooked pumpkin or squash
- ½ cup honey or maple syrup
  pinch salt
- 1½ cups water
- 2 tablespoons apple juice
- 1 teaspoon ground cinnamon
- ½ teaspoon fresh grated ginger
- ½ teaspoon ground nutmeg
- 1 teaspoon alcohol-free vanilla extract (see pp. 59–60)
- ½ cup cubed tofu or 2 tablespoons arrowroot plus 2 table-spoons tahini

To prepare crust: preheat oven to 350°F. Grind almonds into powder in dry blender, then do the same with walnuts. In a bowl, mix nuts with rest of ingredients and press into nine-inch pie dish. Bake 10 minutes. Let cool while mixing pie filling. *Makes one crust.*

To make filling: Preheat oven to 350°F. In blender, blend pumpkin or squash until creamy. Add remaining ingredients to blender. Blend well and pour into pie crust. Bake 45 minutes. *Fills one large nine-inch pie.*

RICE DREAM ICE CREAM OR SORBET

Both of these frozen desserts can be purchased at a health food store. Rice Dream is an ice cream substitute that comes in many flavors. Vanilla or carob are flavors that contain ingredients acceptable for the Simplification Phase. Make sure you read the ingredients for any of the other flavors, as they may include corn oil or cocoa.

Their Sorbet is a sherbet substitute made from fruit juices only. All flavors are delicious, but you should avoid the citrus flavors while on this diet.

A fun topping for Rice Dream or Sorbet is granola or roasted, chopped nuts.

TAHINI CUSTARD

    3   medium-size sweet apples, peeled and sliced
  3½   cups water
   ½   cup maple syrup or honey
   ½   teaspoon salt
    3   tablespoons tahini
    2   packages plain gelatin or 5 tablespoons agar-agar flakes*

Garnish:
    1   kiwi fruit, sliced

Mix all ingredients, except kiwi fruit, together in a saucepan. Bring to a boil, reduce flame to low, and simmer, covered, for 3 minutes. Remove from heat and let cool. Place in a blender and blend until smooth and creamy. Pour into dish or individual cups. Chill. Garnish with kiwi fruit before serving. *Serves 4.*

*Agar-agar flakes can be purchased at a health food store.

RECIPES FOR THE CHALLENGE PHASE

This section contains a few recipe ideas to help you reintroduce corn and yeast-free wheat. We have included recipes for these two food groups only because it is sometimes difficult to find recipes that include these foods without other ingredients that have not yet been reintroduced. You'll find the other foods easy to reintroduce since they involve simple and widely used foods such as eggs, oranges, and breads.

Corn Challenge Recipes

- Quick Corn Bread
- Cornmeal Mush

Yeast-free Wheat Challenge Recipes

- Blueberry Muffins
- Blueberry Pancakes
- Cranberry Bread
- Pumpkin-Nut Muffins

QUICK CORN BREAD

	soy margarine or olive oil
2	cups cornmeal
1	cup rice flour or rye flour
½	teaspoon salt
1¼	teaspoons baking soda
2	tablespoons arrowroot
2	tablespoons sesame or corn oil
2	tablespoons honey
2	cups water

Preheat oven to 400°F. Grease a nine-inch-square baking dish with soy margarine or olive oil. Mix dry ingredients together in bowl, then mix wet ingredients and add to dry, stirring just until mixed in. Pour into baking dish. Bake 20–30 minutes, until golden brown and top springs back when touched.

CORNMEAL MUSH

	½ cup cornmeal (*not* enriched; available at health food store if not at supermarket)
	pinch salt
1	cup boiling water
	maple syrup or honey (optional)

Stir cornmeal and salt into boiling water. Cover, turn heat to low, and simmer for 20 minutes. Serve as is or topped with maple syrup or honey. *Serves 1–2.*

BLUEBERRY MUFFINS

         soy margarine or olive oil
     2   cups rolled oats
     2   cups whole wheat pastry flour*
     1   teaspoon baking soda
     ½   teaspoon salt
     1½ cups water
     1   tablespoon olive oil
     2   tablespoons honey
     ½   cup fresh or frozen blueberries (no sugar added)

Preheat oven to 400°F. Grease muffin tins with soy margarine or
olive oil. Mix ingredients together in order given. Fill muffin tins
three-quarters full with batter. Bake for 20 minutes, until muffins
are golden brown and spring back when touched. *Makes 1½ dozen.*

*Available at health food stores.

BLUEBERRY PANCAKES

     3   cups whole wheat flour
     1½ teaspoons baking soda
     1   teaspoon salt
     2   egg equivalents (see p. 56)
     1   tablespoon olive oil
     2½ cups water
     1   cup fresh or frozen blueberries (no sugar added)
         olive oil

Mix ingredients together in bowl in order given. Drop onto pre-
heated skillet greased with olive oil. Fry until golden brown. *Makes
12 pancakes.*

CRANBERRY BREAD

         olive oil
         whole wheat flour
     2   cups whole wheat or whole wheat pastry flour*
     2   cups unbleached white or whole wheat pastry flour*

  1 tablespoon corn-free baking powder (see p. 54)
  1 teaspoon baking soda
  1 teaspoon salt
  ½ teaspoon ground cinnamon
  ¼ teaspoon ground nutmeg
  ½ cup sesame or soy oil
  1¼ cups maple syrup
  1¼ cups water
  2 cups fresh or frozen cranberries
  1 cup chopped nuts

Preheat oven to 350°F. Grease two 9 × 3 × 5-inch bread pans with olive oil and dust with whole wheat flour. Sift or mix dry ingredients together. Blend oil, maple syrup, and water and add to dry ingredients. Mix just to moisten. Fold in cranberries and nuts. Pour into loaf pans. Bake 55–60 minutes. Cool. (This bread will slice better the next day.) *Makes 2 loaves.*

*Available at health food stores.

PUMPKIN-NUT MUFFINS

       olive oil
  1 cup walnuts, chopped
  1½ cups whole wheat or whole wheat pastry flour*
  ½ teaspoon salt (optional)
  ½ teaspoon ground cinnamon
  ½ teaspoon ground nutmeg
  1 teaspoon corn-free baking powder (see p. 54)
  1 teaspoon baking soda
  ¼ cup honey
  ¼ cup sesame oil
  1 egg equivalent (see p. 56)
  ½ cup water
  1 cup finely grated pumpkin or canned pumpkin

Preheat oven to 250°F. Grease muffin tin with olive oil. Chop walnuts and place in dry baking pan. Roast walnuts for 10–15 minutes, until aromatic. Remove from oven and raise temperature to 400°F.

*Available at health food stores.

Combine flour, salt, cinnamon, nutmeg, baking powder, and baking soda. In another bowl, blend honey, oil, egg equivalent, and water. Add roasted walnuts and pumpkin. Cut in flour mixture with a pastry blender or spoon just until mixed. (This makes a lighter muffin than if beaten together.) Fill muffin tin three-quarters full with batter. Bake approximately 20 minutes, until muffins are golden brown and spring back when touched. *Makes 12 muffins.*

MEAL SCHEDULE PLAN FOR THE SIMPLIFICATION PHASE

Use this meal schedule to combine your own ideas with recipes included in this book to help you create a week of delicious meals.

	First Day Date ____	Second Day Date ____	Third Day Date ____	Fourth Day Date ____
Morning Meal				
Morning Snack				
Noon Meal				
Afternoon Snack				
Evening Meal				
Evening Snack				

	Fifth Day Date _____	Sixth Day Date _____	Seventh Day Date _____

5 · Dietary Supplements

We have already seen that due to weakened immune systems, the number of people suffering from food allergies has increased as the nutritional quality of our diets has decreased. It appears obvious that one way to lessen the severity of allergic attacks, or even to rid yourself completely of the allergy, is to build up your immune system. This is not a fast process; it may take months or years, but it can be done. The best way to begin is by eating highly nutritious, varied, and well-balanced meals made from fresh foods. For many people, however, this is very difficult given the hurried life-styles that make them feel dependent on processed foods. If you are one of these individuals, you may want to help strengthen your immune system with vitamin and mineral supplements, but only after you have completed the Simplification Diet Program.

Although we believe that it is useful to supplement your diet, particularly with the antioxidant vitamins E, C, and beta carotene (the vegetable form of vitamin A), it is difficult to give specific recommendations in a general book of this type. Everyone's nutrient requirements differ as does dietary intake. The way we approach this dilemma is with general recommendations for safe and useful total daily vitamin and mineral intake. These amounts include both the vitamins and minerals present in the foods you eat in addition to any supplements. Use the chart below as a guide for taking supplements.

The most rational way to take supplements is first to determine

**Total Recommended Daily Qualities of Nutrients
(Combined Amount in Foods and Supplements)**

Nutrient	Amount
Calcium	1,200–1,800 mg
Magnesium	600–900 mg
Vitamin C	1,000–3,000 mg
Bioflavonoids	1,000–3,000 mg
Thiamine (vitamin B_1)	10–100 mg
Riboflavin (vitamin B_2)	10–100 mg
Niacin (vitamin B_3)	10–100 mg
Pantothenic acid (vitamin B_5)	50–250 mg
Pyridoxine (vitamin B_6)	20–100 mg
Vitamin B_{12}	50–200 mcg
Biotin	200–600 mcg
Folic acid	400–800 mcg
Vitamin A	5,000–15,000 IU
Beta carotene (vegetable vitamin A)	20,000–40,000 IU
Vitamin D*	0–100 IU
Vitamin E	200–600 IU
Iron†	10–30 mg
Copper	3–6 mg
Zinc	20–50 mg
Manganese	10–20 mg
Chromium	100–200 mcg
Selenium	100–200 mcg
Iodine	150–300 mcg

IU = International Units   mcg = microgram (one millionth of a gram)
mg = milligram (one thousandth of a gram)

*Vitamin D is potentially toxic and should not be taken by most people. The exceptions are individuals who are chronically indoors, such as the elderly, who should perhaps receive up to 100 IU of vitamin D per day. Your doctor can do a simple blood test to see if you need a vitamin D supplement.

†Iron supplements should not be taken indiscriminately. Those with arthritis symptoms and other allergic diseases may aggravate their problems if they take supplements containing iron. Iron is necessary for a healthy immune system, but in just the right amounts. If a need for iron supplements is indicated by blood tests, then they should be used. Serum ferritin, measured by a blood test, generally is accepted as a good indication of your iron status. Your doctor can order this test from any clinical laboratory.

how much nutrition you are getting from your daily food, then determine what quantity of nutrition is optimal, calculate the difference, and make it up first by increasing the quality of your foods and then by adding supplements. To discover the nutrient value of your foods, you can check *Bowes and Church's Food Values of Portions Commonly Used* by J. A. T. Pennington and N. H. Church (see Bibliography), a standard reference available in most libraries and bookstores, or you can use any one of the inexpensive diet analysis programs available for use on home computers. Call your local computer store and ask about this software.

If you don't want to go through all the trouble of figuring out your dietary intake, you can simply take a high-dose multiple supplement that contains at least 1,000 mg of vitamin C, 15 mg (15,000 IU) of beta carotene, 200 IU of vitamin E, and 20 mg of zinc (with 3 mg of copper to balance the zinc). Use the chart on p. 111 for general guidelines.

In addition to the vitamins and minerals given in the chart, we recommend essential fatty acids. Until recently, researchers thought there was only one major type of essential fatty acid, the kind found in corn, peanut oil, other Southern oils, meats, and dairy products (the omega-6 oils).

We now know of another type of essential fatty acid, alpha-linolenic acid (omega-3 oils), found in large quantities only in fish oils and walnut, soy, and linseed (flaxseed) oils. These oils are essential to good health. They have been shown to reduce inflammatory allergic conditions and to help skin problems such as eczema.

Linseed oil (available in health food stores) contains a very high amount of this "new" type of omega-3 essential fatty acid. One teaspoon to two tablespoons per day is the recommended dosage.

An easy way to get this fatty acid into your diet is to eat one salad per day with a linseed oil dressing. Mix the following for a delicious new salad dressing:

    1 cup linseed oil
    ½ cup vinegar
    1 tablespoon tamari
    1 tablespoon crushed dried basil

Please note that this dressing contains yeast products (tamari and vinegar). If you have a yeast allergy, substitute linseed oil for olive oil in the salad dressings listed on pages 58–59. Be absolutely sure to buy food-grade linseed oil in a health food store, and not the type of linseed oil sold in a hardware store. You must refrigerate this oil to prevent it from becoming rancid. It is helpful to add the contents of a vitamin E capsule (400 IU) to the bottle of oil to prevent rancidity. For this purpose, it is best to use vitamin E labeled "Tocopherol" and not the ones labeled "Tocopheryl Acetate" or "Tocopheryl Succinate."

Consider these supplement suggestions *after* you finish the Simplification Diet Program. *It is important to remember that you cannot take any supplements during the Simplification Diet Program.* In our experience, some individuals will react to the most unlikely supplements. We had one case in which a person reacted to plain magnesium oxide powder, as pure and innocuous as it is. There is no way to absolutely predict what your reactivities will be and which supplements may cause a reaction in your body.

After you have completed the Simplification Diet Program, add the supplements you want to take one at a time, just as if they were the foods you reintroduced in the Challenge Phase. Wait two days before introducing another to make sure you have no allergic reaction to that particular supplement. Remember, many commercially produced vitamin and mineral supplements can in themselves cause allergy problems. This is particularly true if the supplements are in tablet form because various ingredients are used to hold the tablets together. Capsules are less likely to cause an allergy problem.

You may also want to take digestive supplements that can help you better digest your problem food, thereby reducing or avoiding an allergic reaction. These digestive supplements fall into four categories:

1. *Stomach acid replacements.* Old-fashioned liquid hydrochloric acid taken through a glass straw is no longer used as a stomach acid replacement. Instead, individuals now take tablets or capsules with the most common active ingredient, either glutamic hydrochloride or betaine hydrochloride. Our stomachs produce hydrochloric acid in response to every meal. Even though there is no truly average meal or average person a good rule of thumb is that most people secrete in the neighborhood of 40 to 50 grains of hydrochloric acid to digest a medium to large meal.

Obviously, too much stomach acid can cause digestive problems:

it can irritate your stomach and esophagus, and interfere with the absorption of your problem food. One good way to determine if you would benefit from hydrochloric acid supplements is to have your doctor measure your stomach acid secretion. Increasing numbers of nutritionally oriented physicians are incorporating the equipment necessary for these tests right into their office practices.

If this type of test is not available, Jonathan Wright, M.D., recommends in his book, *Dr. Wright's Book of Nutritional Therapy,* that you take betaine hydrochloride or glutamic hydrochloride (available at most health food stores) on three consecutive mornings, taking one capsule on the first day, two capsules on the second day, and three capsules on the third day. The capsules should be taken first thing in the morning on an empty stomach. If you have no adverse reaction, you may then take 5 to 30 grains (one grain equals approximately 65 mg) with each meal for a week, building up gradually, and see how your digestion changes. If your digestion improves, with less gas or indigestion, it is usually an indication that your stomach has not been producing enough acid for proper digestion.

If you have a bad reaction, which means anything that hurts or feels bad—heartburn, increased gas, or stomach pains—by all means stop taking the hydrochloric acid. In fact, you can actually neutralize the acid by taking baking soda (sodium bicarbonate) in water or stomach antacid tablets such as Tums (have them on hand). Remember that the amount needed by individuals can vary widely and the best way to determine how much you need is to consult your physician.

2. *Pancreatic enzymes.* These are tablets or capsules of pancreatic enzymes that pose less of a potential problem than taking stomach acid supplements. The quality of these products varies greatly, however, and the only practical way for you to find out if they are helping is if you have improved digestion, usually indicated by reduced gas, bloating, and cramping.

3. *Fiber powders.* These products can be useful in increasing the speed at which digested food moves through your intestines. The fiber supplements which are most useful and least likely to cause allergic reactions are powdered psyllium husks and oat bran. Oat bran can be bought as is, or under the brand name Mothers Oats (a hot breakfast cereal) at health food stores. Powdered psyllium

husks (with no sugar added) can be found generically labeled in most pharmacies, sold under common brand names such as Metamucil (check to see it has no sugar or flavorings), or the Yerba Prima brand at health stores.

4. *Lactobacillus acidophilus preparations.* Lactobacillus acidophilus are one type of "good bacteria" in our intestines, and we most commonly ingest these bacteria by eating yogurt. It has been estimated that there are four pounds of bacteria in the human digestive tract! These bacteria play an important role in digesting food, as well as producing such important nutrients as vitamin B_{12}, which we absorb and use.

If you have a dairy allergy, use dairy-free Lactobacillus acidophilus preparations. The powders are usually more potent than tablets or capsules. Dosage of ½ teaspoon of powder mixed in water or juice twice a day for a few weeks, along with a high-fiber diet, is often helpful for aiding digestion and preventing gas.

If you use any of these supplements, read the labels carefully. Be sure to purchase only supplements that do not contain other ingredients, such as sugar, mixed in with them.

As we stated earlier, finding your problem food is only half the battle. Once that is accomplished you have the job of creating a new diet that will bring you good health and vitality. Often, supplements can help you to do this.

6 · Problems and Solutions

There are a few minor problems that could sabotage your effort to faithfully follow the Simplification Diet Program. This chapter will examine these problems and offer some solutions. We hope that knowing in advance what kind of ruts might be on the road ahead will keep you from stumbling.

BROKEN DIET

The most common problem is the broken diet. If you eat a "forbidden" food during the Simplification or Challenge Phase, you may be thrown in the wrong direction and end up with false results. It's very important to follow the diet strictly from beginning to end. What should you do if you slip? Mike's story will explain.

Mike called my office late one evening after successfully completing five of the seven days of the Simplification Diet. He explained that he had invited a friend to his house for dinner. He didn't want to discuss his food problem with her just yet, and he didn't want to risk eating out, so a home-cooked meal seemed like the perfect solution. He was halfway through his salad when he realized that while he was in the kitchen, his friend must have put the prepared salad dressing (which he had left out for her) on his salad as well. "What should I do?" he asked. "It was only a little bit, but I do have a headache."

My answer to Mike, and to you if you slip, is one with good news and bad news. The good news is that you have learned something about the relationship between the food you ate and your physical symptoms—the ultimate goal of this program. And you should keep in mind that no one is angry with you. It takes many people more than one try to get on track and successfully complete the program, but they do it. You can, too. It's also good to know that all is not lost; you don't "ruin everything" by making a mistake. You simply lose a bit of time.

The bad news is that you can't make "one little slip," pretend it didn't happen, and just keep going along on the diet. If you eat an eliminated food during the Simplification Phase and suffer a return of your symptoms, you must go back to the Simplification Diet and follow it strictly until the symptoms cease. This can take anywhere from one to ten days, depending on the severity of the reaction. When the symptoms have stopped completely, continue the Simplification Phase for two more days and then go on to the Challenge Phase.

If you eat a food during the Challenge Phase that shouldn't have been reintroduced yet and have an adverse reaction, you won't know if the cause is the food you intentionally reintroduced or the one you ate by mistake. If this happens to you, back up to the food group you reintroduced before your slip. Stay there until your symptoms cease, then go ahead with the program.

If, during either the Simplification Phase or the Challenge Phase, you eat a food you were not supposed to eat, but feel no adverse reaction, don't assume you aren't allergic to that food and reintroduce it to your diet. You may not have eaten enough to bring your sensitivity level over its threshold and experience symptoms. It's impossible to be sure. If this happens, talk nicely to yourself, strengthen your commitment to complete the program, and immediately get back on the diet at the same spot you fell off. You may feel badly because you lost some resolve, but in this case no harm is done and you haven't lost any time.

People break the Simplification Phase and/or Challenge Phase of this diet for many reasons, but we have found three reasons mentioned over and over again.

One common reason is that many people attempt to take on the program at the wrong time. It doesn't make much sense, for example, to start on December 15, just before the holiday season in which food is a major part of the festivities. You also don't want to begin two days before a big family celebration or a food-centered event. Timing is important, so pick a thirty-day period that is relatively free of food-centered social obligations or major life stresses. This will make your job much easier and increase your chance for success.

Another reason people break the diet is that they have not taken allowable foods with them when they are away from home. It is very important not to get in a situation where you are ravenous and feel like you have to eat something right away, no matter what it is. In this situation you're bound for failure. Both of these problems can be avoided by planning ahead.

The third reason is the belief that eating a tiny bit of an eliminated food won't make any difference. This simply isn't true. It's hard to imagine how the body can react to a small morsel of food, but think for a moment how a tetanus or other vaccine works. To become vaccinated against tetanus, your doctor injects you with a tiny amount of the tetanus antigen. The idea is that when you are vaccinated with tetanus, your body develops an immune memory which aids in fighting against future infection. This is accomplished with an injection of the tetanus protein that is so small it is hard to measure without very sensitive laboratory instruments. The vast bulk of the injection is simply a carrier fluid.

In the same way, when you eat "only a tiny bit" of a food to which you are sensitive, your body's immune system may respond with a full-blown reaction.

To complete the Simplification Diet Program successfully you must be very strict about eliminating the foods from your diet that need to be avoided.

DIGESTIVE PROBLEMS

The following are some digestive problems associated with the Simplification Diet Program.

1. *Gas.* It is possible that as you progress through the Simplification Diet, you may experience excessive gas (although some find

that their gas problem is solved by this diet!). If your gas increases it usually means you are eating more high-fiber foods than before, such as brown rice and oats, as well as vegetables. Don't worry about a little extra gas, but if you are uncomfortable and want to get rid of it without breaking the Simplification Diet, purchase some activated charcoal tablets at your local pharmacy or health food store. Taking a few charcoal tablets after each meal for a few days usually solves the problem. Be sure, however, that the tablets contain nothing but charcoal so they don't introduce an unwanted substance into your diet. You certainly don't want to add anything you may be allergic to in the form of vitamins, drugs, or any other kind of tablets.

2. *Constipation.* If you find after a few days on the Simplification Diet that you are constipated, it is usually because your system is slow to adjust to the new diet. If this happens, increase your liquid intake (especially water) to six to eight glasses each day. You should also increase the amount of fiber in the Simplification Diet by consuming more of the allowable raw vegetables and cooked grains.

3. *Diarrhea.* If you develop diarrhea while on the Simplification Diet, you should suspect one of the new foods you have introduced to your system as the cause. Look back at your food diary to see if there is any connection between a new food and the onset of the diarrhea. If there is, stop eating that food completely and continue with the rest of the diet phase.

If you can't find any cause for the diarrhea, and it is severe and lasts for more than two days, stop the Simplification Diet and see your doctor. There is something else going on with your digestive system at this time and it's not a good idea to continue with this change in your diet.

HUNGER

If you find that you're hungry all the time, it's probably because you don't know exactly what you are allowed to eat. Go over the list on pages 34–35, and make sure you have plenty of the foods you like on hand. Eat as much of them as you want. Then reread chapter four for help in planning your meals. You can also make up snack bags to carry with you so you won't be caught hungry away from home with nothing to eat.

WITHDRAWAL

It is very common on the Simplification Diet Program to actually feel worse before you feel better. If you experience a downtrend and actually feel worse around the third or fourth day, this is not unusual (as long as you are not jeopardizing your own safety with a dangerous health problem such as escalating asthma attacks). If you experience a simple problem such as fatigue, grit your teeth, stick with the program, and do not give up. You are feeling the effects of withdrawal. Many people report that at the end of the first week they feel much better.

However, if your symptoms don't improve, it could be because you are reacting to one of the new foods in your diet. Look back at your food diary to see if there is any connection between a new food and your symptoms. For instance, you may be eating more nuts or soy products on the Simplification Diet than you used to eat. You should suspect soy as the culprit if you can see in your food diary that every time you put soy milk on your cereal in the morning, you got the same adverse reaction. If this happens, try eliminating soy. You should feel much better within two to three days if you have identified the right food. This means that you will have to extend the Simplification Phase of the diet a few days until you are truly symptom-free.

EATING AWAY FROM HOME

You have to do a lot of advance planning if you dine out or travel during the Simplification Diet Program, but it certainly can be done.

The easiest way to handle meals away from home is to "brown bag" it. Remember, this is a limited period of time for detective work, not a long-term commitment to the requirements of the Simplification Diet Program. Take as much food with you as possible. For example:

- raw almonds (these nuts keep the longest)
- wheat-free granola (make sure it contains no mixed-vegetable or corn oil)
- soy milk in the little pouches that don't need refrigeration
- cans of tuna fish
- homemade Rice Balls rolled in toasted sesame seeds (see p. 70)
- raw carrots
- raw celery
- raw green peppers
- fresh fruit
- Wasa Lite Rye Crackers

If you're going to bring your lunch to work, you can make it after dinner each night with any leftovers. A great method is to use a round Tupperware or Rubbermaid bowl-like container. These are airtight and will keep your lunch fresh and neat. Pack leftover rice, steamed vegetables, leftover beans, or fish or chicken on top of your leftover salad. Dribble a bit of a substitution salad dressing down the side: if you don't soak the whole salad, it won't get soggy. Replace the lid and store the container in the refrigerator overnight. The next morning you're all set for lunch.

You can also eat at a restaurant if you plan ahead so you will order only allowable foods. The safest breakfast menu is oatmeal and a fresh fruit salad. For lunch or dinner you can order broiled fish or chicken, a vegetable without butter, a "dry" salad with plain olive oil on the side, and a baked potato. Many restaurants also have a salad bar which makes it easy to choose allowable foods. Just be careful to stay away from cold salad mixtures (like bean salads) and marinated vegetables—they're usually made with vinegar.

Eating away from home does make it a bit harder to follow the Simplification Diet Program, but not impossible. These circumstances just give you one more additional challenge: Plan ahead!

FOOD CONFUSION

Don't let yourself become overwhelmed worrying about what's an "okay" food and what's "forbidden." You have three simple guidelines to help you. Refer to them whenever you're confused.

1. Eat mostly single-ingredient fresh foods.

2. Read all food labels very carefully. Never assume anything. Companies often change the ingredients from one month to the next.

3. Don't guess or experiment. Stick with the food and menu suggestions listed in this book and you can't go wrong.

NO RELIEF FROM SYMPTOMS

There are two reasons why you might not feel any relief from your symptoms even after fourteen days on the Simplification Diet:

1. There is a very rare group of people who have a food allergy yet show no sign of relief on this diet. This may occur if you have an unusual sensitivity to a food not included in the simplification list of problem foods. If this happens to you, there is another simplification diet that follows the same process as the Simplification Diet Program, but it eliminates more foods from your diet. At this point, however, food allergy detection is no longer a self-help situation. You need to contact a professional nutritionist or a medical doctor who is familiar with and supportive of simplification diets. He or she will give you a new list of additional foods to eliminate from your diet, as well as suggested meal plans that can be prepared with the remaining allowable foods.

This professional may also want to try laboratory testing at this time. Although the results are not always accurate, there are laboratory methods that can screen large numbers of foods, and the results can then be cross-checked by using the Simplification Diet Program process of clearing the suspected food from your body and then reintroducing it in large quantities for two days. If you do react adversely, you will have found your problem food by combining laboratory tests with the Simplification Diet Program.

2. It could always happen that you do not feel any relief from your symptoms after the Simplification Diet because you do not have a food allergy. Usually this only happens if traditional medical testing and treatment procedures were not tried before beginning the search for a food allergy. This situation is rare because most

people don't even consider the possibility that food allergies could be causing their discomfort until they have exhausted all other possibilities.

OVERREACTION

Although overreaction is a very rare occurrence, there are some people who may have such a severe allergic attack when a problem food is reintroduced into their diets that it is best for them to follow the Simplification Diet Program under medical supervision. This is especially true if you have had severe asthma, laryngeal edema (swelling in the throat), or anaphylaxis (unusually severe allergic reaction which impairs breathing) at any time in the past.

ATTITUDE

This is a health plan, not a method of torture. Keep in mind that the Simplification Diet Program involves carving out one month of your life to help you determine once and for all exactly what foods you may be sensitive to, how these foods make you feel, and how to improve your health by removing these foods from your diet. Although that's a lot of work to do in such a short time, you can do it—especially if you have a positive attitude.

Maintaining a positive attitude throughout this process will be easier if you focus on the foods you can eat. Make sure you figure out which treats are fine to have around, then get rid of any foods that are not included in the diet. You might even view this program as a delightful challenge to your culinary abilities—see what marvelous creations you can conjure up, given the unusual ingredients. Above all, stay positive and never lose sight of why you're doing this program. In the future you'll be very glad you made this small sacrifice.

7 · Food Allergies and Children

DOES MY CHILD HAVE A FOOD ALLERGY?

Children who suffer chronic ailments for no apparent medical reason, or who have been labeled hyperactive or hyperkinetic, may actually be ill or "acting up" because of food allergies. Dr. Doris Rapp, pediatrician and clinical assistant professor of pediatrics at the state University of New York at Buffalo and author of *Allergies and the Hyperactive Child,* has created an excellent checklist to help you identify symptoms in your child that might be related to a food allergy. Look over the following common and atypical symptoms of food allergies and see how many apply to your child. The more symptoms you check off, the more likely your child is allergic to something he is eating.

POSSIBLE COMMON SYMPTOMS OF ALLERGY

Eye Allergy

puffy eyes? _____

wrinkles under eyes? _____

black circles under eyes? _____

itchy eyes? _____

red eyes? _____

watery eyes? _____

both eyes affected? _____

burning eyes? _____

painful eyes? _____

eyes light sensitive? _____

Nose Allergy

(When noting nose allergy symptoms, try also to keep track of how often they occur.)

stuffy nose? _____

watery, runny nose? _____

sneezes several times in a row? _____

rubs nose upwards? _____

wiggles nose? _____

picks nose? _____

clears throat often? _____

has one cold after another, but not sick? _____

   how often per month? _____

   other times? _____

nose bleeds? _____

   how often? _____

Chest Allergy

wheeze or asthma? _____

   with infection? _____

   other times? _____

cough or wheeze? _____

  with laughter? _____

  with exercise? _____

  with cold air? _____

  with cold drinks? _____

  at night? _____

  when it's damp outside? _____

Skin Allergy

eczema or atopic dermatitis? _____

itchy rash in arm or leg creases? _____

hives or welts? _____

itchy skin, no rash? _____

itchy rash on body? _____

cracked toenails or fingernails? _____

POSSIBLE ATYPICAL SYMPTOMS OF ALLERGY

Ear Allergy

recurrent fluid behind eardrums? _____

on and off hearing trouble? _____

ear popping? _____

flushed, red earlobes? _____

ringing in ears? _____

dizziness? _____

Intestinal Allergy

colic over age 6 months when infant? _____

unable to drink milk as infant? _____

swelling of face or lips? _____

soreness at edges of lips? _____

irritation at corners of mouth? _____

excess drooling? _____

mottled "bald" patches on tongue? _____

deep grooves or fissures in tongue? _____

excessive throat mucus? _____

itchy roof of mouth? _____

canker sores (ulcers on gums, inside cheeks)? _____

bad breath? _____

clucking throat sounds? _____

frequent nausea? _____

frequent stomachaches? _____

excess stomach gas? _____

bloated stomach? _____

frequent diarrhea? _____

frequent constipation? _____

itchy rectal area? _____

ulcers, gastric or peptic? _____

colitis? _____

Nervous System

constant wiggling about? _____

irritable? _____

hyperactive, restless? _____

clumsy? _____

listless, tired? _____

hostile, fights a lot? _____

cries often or easily? _____

unhappy? _____

behavior problems? _____

seems "spaced-out"? _____

talks nonsense? _____

talks too much? _____

sleeps poorly? _____

nightmares? _____

sleepy and tired in morning? _____

sleepy after eating? _____

sleepy after napping? _____

unexplained depression? _____

seizures? _____

stutters? _____

good vocabulary but can't read? _____

can't draw, print, or write? _____

can't concentrate or poor attention span? _____

dislikes loud noises? _____

dislikes bright lights? _____

dislikes many odors? _____

Skin Allergy

easily bruised? _____

tender, sore skin spots? _____

swollen face or feet? _____

puffy fingers or hands? _____

Urinary Problems: Bladder or Kidney

wets pants in daytime? _____

wets bed at night? _____

   how many times per week? _____

   how many times per month? _____

recurrent bladder infections? _____

other kidney or bladder problems? _____

needs to urinate at night? _____

pain with urination? _____

frequent need to urinate during the day? _____

blood in urine? _____

burning when passing urine? _____

needs to rush to urinate? _____

do urine problems recur at specific times each year? _____

Miscellaneous

headaches? _____

growing pains? _____

muscle aches? _____

pain in neck or shoulder? _____

backaches? _____

leg cramps? _____

joint aches? _____

tingling in arms and legs? _____

excessive perspiration? _____

oversensitive to cold? _____

excessive infections? _____

frequent fevers without infections? _____

vaginal itching or irritation? _____

irregular heartbeat? _____

sudden rapid heartbeat? _____

In addition to this checklist, a child's face often tells the whole story. If he looks pale and washed out or has dark circles under the eyes, a chronic runny nose, or creases under the eyes, chances are your child is reacting to a food. In babies, mothers will often see patches of red skin on the cheeks, a ridge of dry skin along the lip line of the upper lip, colic, or what has been termed the "burned butt syndrome," a rash on the buttocks that is so raw and red it looks like a burn.

One recent study showed that one-third of the colicky breastfed babies studied were reacting to the cow's milk present in their mother's diet. When the mothers eliminated milk products, the colic disappeared in their babies. Other foods in the mother's diet such as wheat, citrus, or corn can also be the culprit in colic.

THE SIMPLIFICATION DIET PROGRAM FOR CHILDREN

Just as it is for adults, the Simplification Diet Program is an appropriate tool for getting to the source of chronic unexplained symptoms. There are no changes or adjustments in the diet program when it is used with a child, but there are a few additional strategies that will make it easier for both parents and child to complete the program successfully. Most important is to prepare the child in advance. Talk to him if he is old enough (at least three years old) about his symptoms and/or behavior problems. Explain that you think you know how to get rid of these problems, but that he'll have to change his diet for a while. Be sure to emphasize all the tasty treats (see dessert recipes) he'll be able to eat, and all the meals that won't change at all (chicken, fish, or beef for dinner, for example, with vegetables, potato and salad). Be positive. Present the program as a fun experiment that you will do together to find the food that causes his allergic reaction.

You might also suggest a reward system. Children tend to be better motivated if they work toward concrete daily goals. One mother with a thirteen-year-old son who loved golf and fishing gave him his choice of either a new golf ball or another lure at the end of each day he successfully completed the Simplification Diet. He had an additional gift awaiting him at the end of the week. This worked well for both the mother and her son.

Younger children often respond well to a gold star chart. Draw up a chart with a space for each meal of every day of the week. Explain to your child that after every meal he successfully completes on the Simplification Diet, he will receive a star. You might even suggest that for every two stars there is another special treat (a trip to the park, a small toy, etc.). Let him know in advance that his efforts to help find his problem food will be rewarded.

Give your child a chance to ask questions and to express his fears and concerns. Be sure all your answers are filled with understanding and that they emphasize the positive. Then, with an open mind, ask your child if he wants to try the diet. If he says no, then let it go. It is crucial that when you ask your child if he is ready to go on the Simplification Diet Program that you are ready and prepared to accept a negative answer. If you allow the child the option of saying no the likelihood of him coming back later and saying, "Yes, now I am ready," is very high. You also must be able to accept that this may not be the best time for your child to tackle this in his mind. It is important to understand this. If your child doesn't want to go on the diet, he won't!

Because it's sometimes worth more to you than to your child to attempt this diet, you may want to offer a very special treat to make it worth your child's effort to do this. Often, if you've figured out the right "carrot" (ask your child; he'll know what he wants!), your child will then be willing to cooperate and give the program an honest try.

Experience shows that very few children will out-and-out refuse this program. Most children don't want to feel ill or uncomfortable. Many are tired of going to doctors or of having teachers and parents yell at them for their behavioral problems. If the program is presented correctly, positively, and with love, they more than likely will respond affirmatively.

Once your child agrees to try the Simplification Diet Program, you still have some advance planning to do. Talk about the program and its goals with all other family members. You will have the greatest chance for success if the entire family follows the Simplification Diet during the meals shared with your child. This is the strongest form of support you can give, and it prevents the child from feeling different from everyone else, or that he is in some way being punished. You might also want to mention your plan to his teacher and to his friends' parents. His teacher can watch to be sure there's no lunch switching going on at school (some schools actually have a "no exchange of lunches" rule), can assist your efforts by not offering him eliminated foods, and can add words of encouragement that will boost his will to succeed.

You can help to ease your child into the diet by slowly removing all eliminated foods from the kitchen. Then let your child help you shop for the new foods you need to stock up on. Let him choose some of the foods and meal plans he wants to try. It is very important that you maintain a sense of fun and excitement by keeping him actively involved in the diet program.

If your child is old enough to write, let him be in charge of the food diary. You will guide his daily entries, of course, but if he is responsible for writing down everything he eats and how he reacts, he will feel like a detective trying to track down the cause of his symptoms—and that's fun!

When the problem food is found, the challenge of keeping that food out of your child's diet begins. But once you've gained his cooperation, you can work together for a healthy and happy future. It's also important to remember that if your child should slip, eat a problem food, and suffer an allergic reaction, at least now you know why he is ill or misbehaving, and you know how to help him get back on the right track. Parent and child both are now in control and that's certainly worth the one month of experimentation it took to get there.

HELPING YOUR CHILD AVOID FOOD ALLERGIES

Of course, it would be best to avoid food allergies right from the beginning, rather than to learn to deal with them once they have appeared. The following information is vital reading for all parents, but it is especially important for those parents who suspect their child might have a predisposition to a food allergy due to the family health history.

Earlier in the book, we discussed the importance of good nutrition in the development of a strong digestive system. Given this information, it is especially important to eat a well-balanced diet during pregnancy, as well as to take a multivitamin/mineral supplement to provide any nutrients that might be lacking in the diet. A well-nourished fetus is less likely to develop food allergies than one that is poorly nourished.

After the baby is born, we strongly recommend that your baby be fed breast milk and only breast milk for the first six months of life. From six months to twelve months, begin to introduce solid food while continuing to breastfeed. The first foods to be introduced should be whole grains such as ground oats, barley, rice, or millet. Then start on yellow vegetables such as winter squash and carrots. It is important that you begin with the yellow vegetables instead of fruits because this will give your baby a taste for less sweet foods. Then introduce yellow fruits such as peaches and apricots. Try to offer mostly seasonal fruits. Rotating foods with the seasons allows for variety and avoids continual, heavy doses of one food, which is often cited as one of the causes of food allergies.

Toward the end of the first year of life, try legumes (dried peas and beans), fish, poultry, and meats. We advise that milk, beef, wheat, corn, citrus, and eggs be introduced after the first birthday to ensure a well-developed intestinal tract and to diminish the chances of becoming reactive to these common foods.

Commercial baby food is never needed if you purchase a baby food grinder at a children's or health food store. You put food into the machine, hand grind it, and end up with ready-to-serve ground food in a little cup that is part of the machine. With a baby-food grinder, it is easy to make two-tablespoon portions. On the other hand, if you try to do this in a blender, you end up throwing out a lot of food because it's difficult to work with such small quantities. The reason we recommend a baby-food grinder is that it is an easy way to feed your baby the freshest, most unadulterated foods possible.

As you introduce foods, give each new food two to three days' trial before moving on to the next. If you see any reactions such as the symptoms listed in the questionnaire in this chapter, stop giving that food, wait until the symptoms clear, and then go on to the next food.

Any food that has already been identified as a problem food for a sibling or parent should not be fed to a baby until the age of twelve to eighteen months, and then slowly introduced in small quantities only. Watch for reactive symptoms. If they do appear, you'll know that this food will probably always be a "high stress" food for your child. This means if very few stresses are present in your child's life (as when there is warm weather, a happy emotional environment, a diet of unprocessed, healthy food, and lots of physical exercise), he can probably tolerate more of that food (perhaps three times a week). But this may not be true if, for example, it is ten degrees below zero outside, the family is going through a divorce, and if the child is eating highly processed foods and getting very little exercise. With circumstances like these present, your child may not be able to tolerate the problem food and you'll notice a recurrence of his allergic reaction.

By feeding your child lots of fresh or frozen vegetables, whole grains, fresh fruits, legumes, fish, and poultry, you will ensure optimum health and increase his chances of avoiding a food allergy.

8 · Living with Food Allergies

What we have given you in this book is a simple method to determine if any of your health problems might be due to a food allergy. This is your tool. More than anything, this tool puts the control in your hands. If your problem is due to a food allergy, then, after completing this program, you will know which food is causing your trouble, and you will be able to control the symptoms.

Finding your food allergies is the "simple and easy" process we promised it would be in chapter one. The more difficult part is accepting your findings and learning to use them to build a healthier future for yourself. This chapter offers suggestions to make this easier for you.

The best way to start living your allergy-free life is to build up the nutritional quality of your diet. As we said in chapter two, because so many American diets are low in essential nutrients, our immune systems are weakened and we are in continual danger of developing food allergies. You can help prevent new allergies from starting, and you can also lessen or even eliminate your present negative response to your problem food, by making a habit of eating a variety of fresh, nutritious foods. Be sure your daily vitamin and mineral intake is adequate (see page 23 for the list of nutrients most often deficient in our diets). Although it takes time and planning to eat properly, it is very important because a strong immune system is your best protection against the distress of food allergies.

When you upgrade the quality of your diet, continue to use your favorite recipes from chapter four in your meal plans. Even after you finish the Simplification Diet Program, they are a valuable collection of nutritious food ideas that will help you in your efforts to avoid the most commonly problematic ingredients. This is also a good time to begin your own recipe collection. Comb books and magazines for nutritious ideas, and don't be afraid to try some food experiments of your own. You're creating a lifetime diet, so try everything that sounds good, is nutritious, and avoids your problem food.

Planning a highly nutritious and well-balanced diet is an important step toward living an allergy-free life. But please also remember to avoid the food that triggers your allergic reaction. This might cause you some confusion if you're allergic to an ingredient that is found in many common foods. To help you stay away from your problem food, and to better find your way around the supermarket and health food stores, we have made up a food shopping chart that you'll find in the appendix. It will guide your selection of common supermarket items, as well as foods that may be new to you and found only in health food stores.

Once you have established a nutritious daily diet, and cleared your body of all traces of your problem food, you might want to try to reintroduce the problem food into your diet. As we explained in chapter three, because everyone's body chemistry is unique, there is no way of predicting how you will react, how much of the food you can eat, or how often you can eat it. You can only find out by experimenting. Also, remember that some allergies are additive, so although you may not be able to tolerate a particular food when your body is stressed by such things as family problems, illness, or air pollen, you may be able to eat it with no problem when these stresses ease.

If you decide to give reintroduction a try, begin with very small amounts once or twice a week, and keep track of any negative reactions. As you increase the amount and the frequency, you'll soon know when you've passed your tolerance threshold because you'll start to feel like you did before you totally eliminated the food from your diet. The recurrence of these symptoms isn't a major problem anymore because now you know what's causing the symptoms and how to eliminate them. You're in control.

The most important factor in determining how successfully you will learn to live with your food allergy is your attitude. Just as a positive and committed attitude is vital to successfully completing the Simplification Diet Program, so is it absolutely necessary in learning to live your allergy-free life.

If you have a food allergy and have learned how to detect and control it, you're a very fortunate person. You're not an invalid or a social outcast; you're just someone who has a negative reaction to a particular food. Some people can't wear wool because it makes them itch, so they don't wear it. Some people can't sit in the sun for too long because it burns their skin, so they don't do it. You can't eat a particular food because you react with negative symptoms, so don't eat it.

This note from one of our clients illustrates our belief that the commitment you make to living on a diet that is best for your health is well worth the effort:

"I don't know why I should find it so astounding that how I feel is largely dependent on what I put into my stomach. Yet it took the process of eliminating and testing foods in my diet to convince me that I didn't have to feel sick all of the time. I am still astounded by how good I feel when I only eat the foods that I am not allergic to."

We hope that through the Simplification Diet Program you, too, will come to this realization and go on to live a vital and healthy life free from the symptoms of food allergies.

Suggested Reading

Borysenko, Joan Z., M.D. *Minding the Body, Mending the Mind.* New York: Addison Wesley, 1987.

Gorden, Thomas. *Parent Effectiveness Training.* New York: New American Library, 1975.

Kaufman, Barry. *To Love is to Be Happy With.* New York: Fawcett Crest, 1977.

Locke, Steven and D. Colligen. *The Healer Within.* New York: E. P. Dutton, 1986.

Nostrand, Carol A. *A Handbook for Improving Your Diet.* 1985.
Send $16.45 check payable to:
Carol A. Nostrand
Eatongude Press
131 West 11th Street
New York, N.Y. 10011
(212) 691-9384

Appendix
Food Shopping

This shopping list will help you find foods that you are allowed to eat during the Simplification Phase, and also after you have identified the food or foods you are allergic to. Each column has a letter corresponding to the food product *not* contained in the item. For example, if a food item does not contain wheat, yeast, and corn, the letters *W, Y,* and *Co* will appear in the column to the right of that food. Each food group is also divided into supermarket and health food store items to help you more easily locate the foods you need.

Since manufacturers sometimes change the ingredients in their foods, always be sure to double-check our listings by reading the ingredient labels on all foods you buy.

Product Does Not Contain

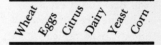

	Wheat	Eggs	Citrus	Dairy	Yeast	Corn

Beverages

Health Food Store Items

	Wheat	Eggs	Citrus	Dairy	Yeast	Corn
Ah Soy (Vanilla)	W	E	Ci	D	Y	
Amazake, *Kendall Food Co.*	W	E	Ci	D	Y	Co
Bambu		E	Ci	D	Y	Co
Cafix	W	E	Ci	D	Y	Co

	Wheat	Eggs	Citrus	Dairy	Yeast	Corn
			Product Does Not Contain			
Cinnamon Apple Spice Tea, *Celestial Seasonings*	W	E	Ci	D	Y	Co
Roma Coffee Substitute, *Natural Touch*	W	E	Ci	D	Y	Co
Soy "M" Milk	W	E	Ci	D	Y	Co
Soy Moo, *Health Valley*	W	E	Ci	D	Y	Co
Sunsoy (Carob)	W	E	Ci	D	Y	Co
Sunsoy (Plain)	W	E	Ci	D	Y	Co

Supermarket Items

	Wheat	Eggs	Citrus	Dairy	Yeast	Corn
V-8 Juice	W	E	Ci	D		Co

Breakfast Cereals

Health Food Store Items

	Wheat	Eggs	Citrus	Dairy	Yeast	Corn
Alpen Cereal, *Weetabix*		E	Ci			
Amaranth Flakes, *Health Valley*	W	E	Ci	D	Y	
Brown Rice Cream, *Erewhon*	W	E	Ci	D	Y	Co
Cream of Rye, *Conagra*	W	E	Ci	D	Y	Co
Crispy Brown Rice	W	E	Ci	D	Y	Co
Fruit-e-o's, *New Morning*	W	E		D	Y	
Golden Oats, *Stow Mills*	W	E	Ci	D	Y	Co
Kashi Breakfast Cereal		E	Ci	D	Y	Co
Oat Bran Flakes, *Health Valley*	W	E	Ci	D	Y	
Oatios, *New Morning* (bagged)		E	Ci	D	Y	Co
Oatios, *New Morning* (boxed)	W	E	Ci	D	Y	Co
Old Fashioned Corn Flakes, *Stow Mills*	W	E	Ci	D	Y	
100% Natural Bran Cereal, *Health Valley*		E	Ci	D		Co

Supermarket Items

	Wheat	Eggs	Citrus	Dairy	Yeast	Corn
Nutri-Grain Almond Raisin Cereal, *Kellogg's*	W	E	Ci	D		
Nutri-Grain Corn Flakes, *Kellogg's*	W	E	Ci	D		
Nutri-Grain Wheat Flakes, *Kellogg's*		E	Ci	D		Co

Product Does Not Contain

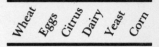

Canned Goods

Health Food Store Items

	Wheat	Eggs	Citrus	Dairy	Yeast	Corn
Mild Vegetarian Chili with Beans, *Health Valley*	W	E	Ci	D		Co
Mild Vegetarian Chili with Lentils, *Health Valley*	W	E	Ci	D	Y	Co
Refried Beans, *Casa Fiesta*	W	E	Ci	D	Y	Co
Spicy Vegetarian Chili with Beans, *Health Valley*	W	E	Ci	D		Co

Supermarket Items

	Wheat	Eggs	Citrus	Dairy	Yeast	Corn
Anchovies, *Empress*	W	E	Ci	D	Y	Co
Bean Sprouts, *La Choy*	W	E	Ci	D	Y	Co
Canadian Sardines in Soya Oil, *Brunswick*	W	E	Ci	D	Y	Co
Granadaisa Sardines, *Durkee*	W	E	Ci	D	Y	Co
Great Northern Beans, *Furman's*	W	E	Ci	D	Y	Co
Kipper Snacks, *King Oscar*	W	E	Ci	D	Y	Co
Pink Salmon, *Chicken of the Sea*	W	E	Ci	D	Y	Co
Premium Chunk White Chicken, *Swanson*	W	E	Ci	D	Y	Co
Red Salmon, *Bumble Bee*	W	E	Ci	D	Y	Co
Sardines, *Geisha*	W	E	Ci	D	Y	Co
Sardines in Tomato Sauce, *Geisha*	W	E	Ci	D	Y	Co
Shrimp, *DeJean's*	W	E	Ci	D	Y	Co
Snow Crab Meat, *Geisha*	W	E	Ci	D	Y	Co
Tiny Cocktail Shrimp, *DeJean's*	W	E	Ci	D	Y	Co
Tuna in water (most brands)	W	E	Ci	D	Y	Co
Water Chestnuts, *Geisha*	W	E	Ci	D	Y	Co
Whole Oysters, *Empress*	W	E	Ci	D	Y	Co

	Wheat	Eggs	Citrus	Dairy	Yeast	Corn
Product Does Not Contain						

Condiments

Health Food Store Items

	Wheat	Eggs	Citrus	Dairy	Yeast	Corn
All Natural Ketchup, *Enrico's*	W	E	Ci	D		Co
Bernard Jensen's Quick Sip	W	E	Ci	D	Y	
Dr. Bronner's Balanced Mineral Bouillion	W	E		D	Y	Co
Hot Cha Cha Texas Salsa	W	E	Ci	D		Co
Mild Salsa Picante, *Enrico's*	W	E	Ci	D		Co
Natural Stoneground Mustard, *Westbrae*	W	E	Ci	D		Co
Taco Seasoning Mix, *Hain*		E	Ci		Y	Co
Unsweetened Un-Ketchup, *Westbrae*	W	E	Ci	D		Co
Wheat Free Tamari Soy Sauce, *San-J*	W	E	Ci	D		Co

Crackers and Chips

Health Food Store Items

	Wheat	Eggs	Citrus	Dairy	Yeast	Corn
Akmak Crackers		E	Ci			Co
All Natural Biscuits (for teethers), *Health Times*	W	E	Ci	D	Y	Co
Arden Rice Cakes (Plain, 5 Grain)	W	E	Ci	D	Y	Co
Corn Chips, *Barbara's*	W	E	Ci	D	Y	
Crispy Cakes (Apple Cinnamon, Natural, Italian Spices)	W	E	Ci	D	Y	Co
French Onion Stoned Wheat Crackers, *Health Valley*		E	Ci	D		Co
Grain Vegetable Stoned Wheat Crackers, *Health Valley*		E	Ci	D		
Herb Stoned Wheat Crackers, *Health Valley*		E	Ci	D		Co
Lundberg Rice Cakes (Brown Rice, Wehani, Mochi, Sweet, Wild Rice)	W	E	Ci	D	Y	Co
Natural Potato Chips, *Barbara's*	W	E	Ci	D	Y	Co
Onion & Garlic Brown Rice Wafers, *Westbrae*	W	E	Ci	D	Y	Co
Rice Chips (Nacho Cheese), *Amsnack*	W	E	Ci		Y	Co
Rice Chips (Onion), *Amsnack*	W	E	Ci	D	Y	Co

Product Does Not Contain

	Wheat	Eggs	Citrus	Dairy	Yeast	Corn
Samurai Puffs, *Westbrae*	W	E	Ci	D		Co
Seaweed Crunch, *Soken*	W	E	Ci	D		
Sesame Brown Rice Wafers, *Westbrae*	W	E	Ci	D		Co
Sesame Stoned Wheat Crackers, *Health Valley*		E	Ci	D		Co
Sesame Wheels, *Soken*		E	Ci	D		Co
Tamari Brown Rice Wafers, *Westbrae*	W	E	Ci	D		Co
Teriyaki Crackers, *San-J*		E	Ci	D		Co
Teriyaki Nuggets, *Edward & Sons*	W	E	Ci	D		Co
Tortilla Chips, *Bearitos*	W	E	Ci	D	Y	
Tortilla Chips, *Mother Earth*	W	E	Ci	D	Y	
Unsalted Brown Rice Wafers, *Westbrae*	W	E	Ci	D	Y	Co
Unsalted Natural Potato Chips, *Barbara's*	W	E	Ci	D	Y	Co
Vegetable Chips, *Soken*	W	E	Ci	D	Y	
Whole Wheat Pretzels, *Barbara's*		E	Ci	D		Co
Yogurt & Green Onion Potato Chips, *Barbara's*	W	E	Ci		Y	Co

Supermarket Items

	Wheat	Eggs	Citrus	Dairy	Yeast	Corn
Kavli Norwegian Crispbread (Thick Style)		E	Ci	D	Y	Co
Kavli Norwegian Crispbread (Thin Style)	W	E	Ci	D	Y	Co
Wasa Crispbread (Lite Rye)	W	E	Ci	D	Y	Co
Whole Wheat Matzos, *Manischewitz*		E	Ci	D	Y	Co

Desserts and Sweet Snacks

Health Food Store Items

	Wheat	Eggs	Citrus	Dairy	Yeast	Corn
Almond Nut Butter Cookies, *Pride o' the Farm*		E	Ci		Y	
Amaranth Cookies, *Health Valley*		E				
Amaranth Graham Crackers, *Health Valley*		E	Ci	D	Y	
Animal Cookies (Cinnamon, Vanilla), *Barbara's*		E	Ci		Y	
Animal Cookies, *Pride o' the Farm*		E	Ci	D	Y	
Banana Cream Nectar Freeze, *Natural Nectar*	W	E	Ci		Y	Co

	Wheat	Eggs	Citrus	Dairy	Yeast	Corn
Product Does Not Contain						
Barley Waffers, *Terra Natural Foods*			Ci			
Betsy's Wild Animal Cookies (Butter Orange)		E			Y	
Brown Rice Baking Mix, *Fearn*	W	E	Ci	D	Y	
Brown Rice & Barley Cookies, *Nature's Warehouse*	W	E	Ci	D		
California Lemon Cookies, *Barbara's*		E			Y	
Carob Coconut Chip Cookies, *Nanak's*	W	E	Ci		Y	
Carob Macaroon, *Jennies of Red Hill Farms*	W		Ci	D	Y	Co
Carob Snaps, *Westbrae*		E	Ci	D	Y	
Cinnamon Candy, *Natural Temptations*	W	E	Ci	D	Y	Co
Coconut Macaroon, *Barbara's*	W		Ci	D		Co
Coconut Macaroon, *Jennies of Red Hill Farms*	W		Ci		Y	Co
Danish Almond Cookies, *Harvest Farm*	W	E	Ci	D	Y	
Dawn's Rice Drops (all flavors)	W	E	Ci	D	Y	Co
Delicious Sesame Crunch, *Barbara's*		E	Ci	D		
Dutch Apple Cookies, *Harvest Farm*	W	E	Ci	D	Y	
Fruit Filled Macaroon, *Jennies of Red Hill Farms*	W			D		Co
Fruit & Nut Cookies, *Barbara's*		E	Ci	D	Y	
Ginger Snaps, *Westbrae*		E	Ci	D		
Glenny's Brown Rice Treat (Peanut & Raisin)	W	E	Ci	D		Co
Glenny's Brown Rice Treat (Plain & Fancy)	W	E	Ci	D	Y	Co
Glenny's Nookies (Almond, Raisin, Coconut, Candy)	W	E	Ci	D		Co
Glenny's Nookies (Sesame)	W	E	Ci	D		Co
Granola Bar (Cinnamon/Oats), *Barbara's*	W	E	Ci	D		Co
Granola Bar (Peanut Butter), *Barbara's*	W	E	Ci	D		Co
Granola Bars (Cinnamon/Raisin), *Nature's Choice*	W	E	Ci			
Granola Bars (Peanut Butter), *Nature's Choice*	W	E	Ci	D		
Honey Grahams, *Midel*		E		D	Y	Co
Ice Bean (Carob, Honey Vanilla)	W	E	Ci	D	Y	Co
Ice Bean (Strawberry)	W	E	Ci	D	Y	
Just Juice Popsicles (Apple, Pineapple, Grape)	W	E	Ci	D	Y	Co

Product Does Not Contain

	Wheat	Eggs	Citrus	Dairy	Yeast	Corn
Maple Waffers, *Terra Natural Foods*			Ci		Y	Co
Nellie Fruit & Nut Sticks	W	E	Ci			
Nouvelle Sorbet (Strawberry)	W	E	Ci	D	Y	Co
Oatmeal Raisin Bar, *Glennys*	W	E	Ci	D		Co
Oatmeal Raisin Cookies, *Barbara's*		E	Ci	D	Y	
Peanut Butter Cookie, *Barbara's*		E	Ci	D		Co
Peanut Butter Snaps, *Westbrae*		E	Ci	D		
Raspberry Cream Nectar Freeze, *Natural Nectar*	W	E	Ci		Y	Co
Rice Dream (Carob Chip)	W	E	Ci	D	Y	
Rice Dream (Lemon)	W	E		D	Y	Co
Rice Dream (Orange)	W	E		D	Y	Co
Rice Dream (Strawberry, Carob, Vanilla)	W	E	Ci	D	Y	Co
Soken Plum Candy		E	Ci	D	Y	Co
Vanilla Ice Bean Sandwiches		E	Ci	D	Y	Co
Whole Wheat Fig Bar, *Marin Brand*		E		D		

Supermarket Items

	Wheat	Eggs	Citrus	Dairy	Yeast	Corn
Dark Sweet Cherries (frozen), *Seabrook*	W	E	Ci	D	Y	Co
Mixed Melon Balls (frozen), *Seabrook*	W	E	Ci	D	Y	Co
Pineapple Chunks in Own Juice, *Dole's*	W	E	Ci	D	Y	Co

Fast Foods

Health Food Store Items

	Wheat	Eggs	Citrus	Dairy	Yeast	Corn
Brown Rice Ramen, *Westbrae*		E	Ci	D		Co
Falafil Mix, *Fantastic Foods*		E	Ci	D		
Frijoles Mix, *Fantastic Foods*	W	E	Ci	D	Y	Co
Japan Pearl Barley Ramen, *Premier*		E	Ci	D		Co
Lentil Pilaf Mix, *Near East*	W	E	Ci	D	Y	Co
Light Links, *Light Foods*			Ci	D		Co
Mushroom Ramen, *Westbrae*		E	Ci	D		Co
Not Dogs, *Soyboy*	W	E	Ci	D	Y	Co
100% Whole Wheat Ramen, *Westbrae*		E	Ci	D		Co

	Wheat	Eggs	Citrus	Dairy	Yeast	Corn
Product Does Not Contain						
Pacific Tempeh Burger, *Soy Deli*	W	E	Ci	D	Y	Co
Soy & Brown Rice Tempeh, *Soyfoods Unlimited*	W	E	Ci	D		Co
Soy Tempeh, *Tempehworks*	W	E	Ci	D		Co
Tabouli Salad Mix, *Fantastic Foods*		E		D	Y	Co
Tempeh Burgers, *Lightlife*	W	E	Ci	D		Co
Three Grain Tempeh, *Tempehworks*	W	E	Ci	D		Co
Tofu Burger Mix, *Fantastic Foods*		E	Ci	D		
Tofu Lasagna, *Legume, Inc.*		E	Ci	D		Co
Tofu Pups, *Lightlife*	W	E	Ci	D		Co
Tofu Scrambler Mix, *Fantastic Foods*		E	Ci	D		Co
Vegetarian Chili Mix, *Fantastic Foods*	W	E		D		
Veggie Burgers, *Mudpie*	W	E	Ci	D	Y	Co
Whole Wheat Macaroni & Cheese, *Westbrae*		E	Ci			Co

Oils and Sweeteners

Health Food Store Items

	Wheat	Eggs	Citrus	Dairy	Yeast	Corn
Barley Malt, *Eden*	W	E	Ci	D	Y	Co
Rice Syrup	W	E	Ci	D	Y	Co

Supermarket Items

	Wheat	Eggs	Citrus	Dairy	Yeast	Corn
100% Pure Vegetable Oil, *Puritan*	W	E	Ci	D	Y	Co
Safflower Oil, *Hollywood*	W	E	Ci	D	Y	Co
Sunflower Oil, *Wesson*	W	E	Ci	D	Y	Co
Sunola Oil	W	E	Ci	D	Y	
Vegetable Oil, *Wesson*	W	E	Ci	D	Y	Co

Pasta

Health Food Store Items

	Wheat	Eggs	Citrus	Dairy	Yeast	Corn
Corn Pasta, *DeBoles*	W	E	Ci	D	Y	
100% Soba, *Mitoku*	W	E	Ci	D	Y	Co
Traditional Soba		E	Ci	D	Y	Co

Product Does Not Contain

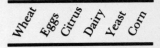

	Wheat	Eggs	Citrus	Dairy	Yeast	Corn
Salad Dressings						
Health Food Store Items						
Fine Herbs Creamy Tofu Dressing, *Nasoya*	W	E	Ci	D		Co
Nasoyanaise, *Nasoya*	W	E	Ci	D		Co
Natural Mayonnaise, *Westbrae*	W			D		Co
Saf-flower Mayonnaise, *Hain*	W			D		Co
Supermarket Items						
Newman's Own Olive Oil & Vinegar Dressing	W	E		D		Co
Sauces						
Health Food Store Items						
Spaghetti Sauce, *Enrico's*	W	E	Ci	D	Y	Co
Supermarket Items						
Aunt Millie's Traditional Meatless Spaghetti Sauce	W	E	Ci			Co
Chunky Homestyle Meatless Spaghetti Sauce, *Prince*	W	E		D	Y	
Natural Applesauce, *Mott's*	W	E	Ci	D	Y	Co
Soups						
Health Food Store Items						
Avgholemono Soup Mix, *Mayacama's*					Y	Co
Black Bean Soup, Dip & Recipe Mix, *Mayacama's*		E	Ci	D	Y	Co
Chicken Broth, *Health Valley*	W	E	Ci	D	Y	Co

	Wheat	Eggs	Citrus	Dairy	Yeast	Corn
					Product Does Not Contain	
Cream of Broccoli Soup Mix, *Mayacama's*					Y	
Cream of Mushroom Soup Mix, *Mayacama's*		E	Ci			Co
Cream of Tomato Soup Mix, *Mayacama's*		E			Y	Co
Creamy Clam Soup Mix, *Mayacama's*		E	Ci		Y	Co
French Onion Soup Mix, *Mayacama's*		E	Ci			Co
Garden Pea Soup Mix, *Mayacama's*	W	E	Ci	D		Co
Instant Miso Soup (Mellow White), *Westbrae*	W	E	Ci	D		Co
Lentil Soup, *Health Valley*	W	E	Ci	D	Y	Co
Lentil Soup Mix, *Mayacama's*		E	Ci			Co
Minestrone Soup, *Hain Naturals*	W	E	Ci	D	Y	Co
Miso-Cup Golden Light, *Edward & Sons*	W	E	Ci	D		Co
Nutra Soup (Vegetable), *Barth's*		E	Ci	D		Co
Potato Leek Soup Mix, *Mayacama's*		E	Ci		Y	Co
Tomato Soup, *Health Valley*	W	E		D	Y	Co
Vegetable Soup, *Health Valley*	W	E	Ci	D	Y	Co
Vegetarian Vegetable Soup, *Hain Naturals*	W	E	Ci	D	Y	
Vegex Bouillion Cubes	W	E	Ci	D	Y	Co

Supermarket Items

	Wheat	Eggs	Citrus	Dairy	Yeast	Corn
Lentil Soup, *Progresso*	W	E	Ci	D	Y	Co
Minestrone Soup, *Progresso*		E	Ci	D	Y	Co

Whole Grains and Whole Grain Products

Health Food Store Items

	Wheat	Eggs	Citrus	Dairy	Yeast	Corn
Essene Bread with Seeds, *Lifestream*		E	Ci	D	Y	Co
Essene Fruit Cake, *Lifestream*		E	Ci	D		Co
Essene Rye Bread with Seeds, *Lifestream*	W	E	Ci	D	Y	Co
Ezekiel 4:9 Sprouted Grain Bread		E	Ci	D		Co
Essene Rye Bread, *Lifestream*	W	E	Ci	D	Y	Co
Food for Life White Rye Bread	W	E	Ci	D		
Garden of Eatin' Corntillas	W	E	Ci	D	Y	
Whole Wheat English Muffins (Cinnamon Raisin), *Matthew's*		E	Ci	D		

	Product Does Not Contain					
	Wheat	*Eggs*	*Citrus*	*Dairy*	*Yeast*	*Corn*
Whole Wheat English Muffins (Plain), *Matthew's*		E	Ci	D		
Whole Wheat Flour Tortillas, *Garden of Eatin'*		E	Ci	D	Y	

Supermarket Items

Kasha, *Wolff's*	W	E	Ci	D	Y	Co
Natural Long Grain Brown Rice, *River*	W	E	Ci	D	Y	Co
Old Fashioned Quaker Oats	W	E	Ci	D	Y	Co
Quick Quaker Oats	W	E	Ci	D	Y	Co

Bibliography

Abba, I. T., 1986. Environmental Illness; A clinical review of 50 cases. *Arch. Intl. Med.* 146:145–149.

Abdulla, M., et al. 1981. Nutrient intake and health status of vegans. Chemical analyses of diets using the duplicate portion sampling technique. *Am. J. Clin. Nutr.* 34:2464–2477.

Adamson, W. B., and Sellers, E. D. 1933. Observations on the incidence of the hypersensitive state in one hundred cases of epilepsy. *J. Allergy* 5:315–326.

Aiuti, F., and Paganelli, R. 1983. Food allergy and gastrointestinal diseases. *Ann. Allergies* 51:275–280.

Alverdy, J., Chi, H. S., and Sheldon, G. F. 1985. The effect of parenteral nutrition on gastrointestinal immunity—the importance of enteral stimulation. *Am. Surg.* 202:681–684.

Anderson, J. A. 1985. Food allergy and food intolerance. *Bol. Assoc. Med. Puerto Rico* 77:215–217.

———. 1985. Food allergy and food intolerance. *J. Dentistry for Children* 52:134–137.

———. 1984. Non Immunologically Mediated Food Sensitivity. *Nutr. Rev.* 42:109–116.

Anderson, J. B., and Lessoff, M. H. 1983. Diagnosis and treatment of food allergies. *Proc. Nutr. Soc.* 42:257–276.

Anderson, R. 1984. The immunostimulatory, anti-inflammatory and anti-allergic properties of ascorbate. *Adv. Nutr. Res.* 19–45.

Atherton, D. J. 1985. Skin disorders and food allergy. *J. Royal Soc. Med.* Suppl. 5:7–10.

Atkins, F. M. 1983. The basis of immediate hypersensitivity reactions to food. *Nutr. Rev.* 41:229–234.

Barbul, A., et al. 1978. White cell involvement in the inflammatory, wound healing, and immune actions of vitamin A. *J. Paren. and Ent. Nutr.* 2:129–138.

Barker, D. J., and Osmond, C. 1986. Infant mortality, childhood nutrition, and ischaemic heart disease in England and Wales. *Lancet* 1077.

Barnes, M. C. 1940. The thyroid in allergy. *Southern Med. J.* 33:1310–1316.

Bartnik, W., and Shorter, R. G. 1985. The immunology of inflammatory bowel disease. *Mater. Med. Pol.* 13:77–84.

Beisel, W. R. 1980. Effects of infection on nutritional status and immunity. *Fed. Proc.* 39:3105–3108.

Beisel, W. R., et al. 1981. Single-nutrient effects on immunologic functions. *JAMA* 245:53–58.

Bellanti, J. A. 1985. *Immunology III*. 2nd ed. Philadelphia: W. B. Saunders.

Bendich, A., Gabriel, E., and Machlin, L. J. 1986. Dietary vitamin E requirement for optimum immune responses in the rat. *J. Nutr.* 116:675–681.

Bentley, S. J., Pearson, D. J. and Rix. 1983. Food hypersensitivity in irritable bowel syndrome. *Lancet* 295–297.

Berman, B. A. 1985. Food allergy. *Cutis* 36:17–19.

Bernstein, M., Day, J. H., and Welsh, A. 1982. Double-blind food challenge in the diagnosis of food sensitivity in the adult. *J. Am. Clin. Immun.* 70:205–210.

Blackwell, B., and Marley, E. 1969. Monoamine oxidase inhibition and intolerance to foodstuffs. *Nutritio et Dieta* 11:96–110.

Block, G., et al. 1985. Nutrient sources in the American diet: quantitative data from the NHANES II Survey. *Am. J. Epidemiol.* 122:27–40.

Bock, S. A. 1983. Food related asthma and basic nutrition. *J. Asthma* 20:377–381.

———. 1980. Food sensitivity—a critical review and practical approach. *Am. J. Dis. Child.* 134:973–982.

———. 1982. The natural history of food sensitivity. *J. Aller. Clin. Immunol.* 69:173–177.

Boissonneault, G. A., and Johnstone, P. V. 1983. Essential fatty acid deficiency, prostoglandin synthesis and humoral immunity in Lewis rats. *J. Nutr.* 113:1187–1194.

Branden, D. L. 1984. Interactions of diet and immunity. *Adv. Exp. Med. Biol.* 177:65–90.

Bray, G. W. 1931. The hypochlorhydria of asthma in childhood. *Quart. J. Med.* 1881–1886.

Breneman, J. C. 1984. *Basics of food allergy*. 2nd ed. Springfield, Mass.: Charles C. Thomas.

———. 1985. Food allergy—a new science. *J. Arkansas Med. Soc.* 81:594–611.

———. 1983. Overview of food allergy: historical perspective. *Ann. Allergy* 51:220–221.

Brown, R. E. 1977. Interaction of nutrition and infection in clinical practice. *Ped. Clin. of N. Am.* 24:241–252.

Buckley, R. H., and Metcalfe, D. 1982. Food allergy. *JAMA* 248:2627–2631.

Buist, R. A. 1983. The malfunctional mucosal barrier and food allergies (editorial). *Intl. Clin. Nutr. Rev.* 3:1–4.

Burke, V. 1972. Gastrointestinal symptoms and cow's milk allergy. *Aust. Paediat. J.* 8:231–232.

Burr, M. L. 1983. Does infant feeding affect the risk of allergy. *Arch. Dis. Child.* 58:561–565.

Businco, L., Benincori, N., and Cantani, A. 1984. Epidemiology, incidence and clinical aspects of food allergy. *Ann. Allergy* 53:615–622.

Cant, A. J. 1985. Food allergy in childhood. *Hum. Nutr.: Appl. Nutr.* 39A:277–293.

Carwin, L. M., and Gordon, R. K. 1982. Vitamin E and immune regulation. *Ann. N.Y. Acad. Sci.* 393:437–451.

Chandra, R. K. 1975. Fetal malnutrition and postnatal immunocompetence. *Am. J. Dis. Child.* 129:450–454.

———. 1981. Immunocompetence as a functional index of nutritional status. *Brit. Med. Bull.* 37:89–94.

———. 1979. Interactions of nutrition, infection and immune response. *Acta. Paed. Scand.* 68:137–144.

———. 1983. Mucosal immune responses in malnutrition. *Ann. N.Y. Acad. Sci.* 409:345–356.

———. 1983. Nutrition, immunity and infection: present knowledge and future directions. *Lancet* 688–691.

———. 1983. Nutrition and immune responses. *Can. J. Physiol.* 61:290–294.

———. 1979. Nutritional deficiency and susceptibility to infection. *Bulletin World Health Organization* 57:167–177.

———. 1980. Nutritional deficiency, immune responses, and infectious illness. *Fed. Proc.* 39:3086–3092.

———. 1984. Parasitic infection, nutrition, and immune response. *Fed. Proc.* 43:251–255.

———. 1980. Single nutrient deficiency and cell-mediated immune responses. *Am. J. Clin. Nutr.* 33:736–738.

———. 1981. Trace elements and immunity: a synopsis of current knowledge. *Food Nutr. Bull.* 3:39–41.

Chandra, R. K., Heresi, G., and Au, B. 1980. Serum thymic factor activity in deficiencies of calories, zinc, vitamin A and pyridoxine. *Clin. Exp. Immunol.* 42:332–335.

Chandra, R. K., and Tejpar, S. 1983. Review diet and immunocompetence.

Int. J. Immunopharmac. 5:175–180.

Cook, G. E., and Joseph, R. 1983. Food allergy and migraine. *Lancet* 1256–1257.

Corman, L. C. 1985. Effects of Specific Nutrients on the Immune Response—Selected Clinical Applications. *Med. Clin. N. Am.* 69:759–790.

———. 1985. The relationship between nutrition, infection, and immunity. *Med. Clin. of N. Am.* 69:519–530.

Coussons, H. W. 1984. Diet and hyperactivity. *J. Ohio State Med. Assoc.* 77:169–73.

Crawford, L. V., and Herrod, H. G. 1981. *Allergy diets for infants.* New York: Year Book Med. Publishers.

Crook, W. G. 1975. Food allergy—the great masquerader. *Ped. Clin. of N. Am.* 22:227–238.

———. 1986. *The Yeast Connection.* 3rd ed. New York: Random House.

———. 1980. *Tracking down hidden food allergy.* Jackson, Tenn.: Professional Books.

Crook, W. G., et al. 1961. Systemic manifestations due to allergy. Report of 50 patients and a review of the literature on the subject (allergic toxemia and the allergic tension-fatigue syndrome). *Pediatrics* 27:791–796.

Cunningham-Rundles, C., et al. 1979. Bovine antigens and the formation of circulating immune complexes in selective immunoglobulin A deficiency. *J. Clin. Invest.* 64:272.

Dalton-Bunnow, M. F. 1985. Review of sulfite sensitivity. *Am. J. Hosp. Pharm.* 42:2220–2226.

Darlington, L. G., Ramsey, N. W., and Mansfield, J. R. 1986. Placebo-controlled, blind study of dietary manipulation therapy in rheumatoid arthritis. *Lancet* 236–238.

Das, M., et al. 1977. Metabolic correlates of immune dysfunction in malnourished children. *Am. J. Clin. Nutr.* 30:1949–1952.

Davenport, H. W. 1982. *Physiology of the digestive tract.* Chicago: Year Book Med. Publishers.

David, T. J. 1984. Anaphylactic shock during elimination diets for severe atopic eczema. *Arch. Dis. in Child.* 59:983–986.

David, T. J., Waddington, E., and Stanton, R. H. 1984. Nutritional hazards of elimination diets in children with atopic eczema. *Arch. Dis. Child.* 59:323–325.

Davison, H. M. 1951. The role of food sensitivity in nasal allergy. *Ann. Allergy* 9:568–572.

Dees, S. C. 1951. Allergic epilepsy. *Ann. Allergy* 9:446–456.

Denman, A. M. 1979. Nature and diagnosis of food allergy. *Proc. Nutr. Soc.* 38:391–402.

Derbes, S. J., and deShazo, R. D. 1985. Urticaria and angioedema: new insights and new entities. *Comp. Ther.* 11:52–59.

deWeck, A. L. 1984. Pathophysiologic mechanisms of allergic and pseudo-allergic reactions to foods, food additives and drugs. *Ann. Allergy* 53:583–586.

Dickerson, J. W. T., and Pepler, F. 1980. Diet and hyperactivity. *J. Hum. Nutr.* 34:167–174.

Dowd, P. S., and Heatley, R. V. 1984. The influence of undernutrition on immunity. *Clin. Sci.* 66:241–248.

Dreizen, S. 1979. Nutrition and the immune response—a review. *Intl. J. Vit. Nutr. Res.* 49:220–228.

Duchateau, J., et al. 1981. Beneficial effects of oral zinc supplementation on the immune response of old people. *Am. J. Med.* 70:1001–1004.

Duke, W. W. 1923. Food allergy as a cause of irritable bladder. *J. Urol.* 10:173–178.

Eaton, K. K. 1982. The incidence of allergy—has it changed? *Clin. Allergy* 12:107–110.

Egger, J., et al. 1985. Hyperkinetic behavior and food sensitivity. *Lancet* 540–545.

Egger, J., et al. 1985. Controlled trial of oligoantigenic treatment in the hyperkinetic syndrome. *Lancet* 540–545.

Egger, J., et al. 1983. Is migraine food allergy? *Lancet* 865–868.

Faulk, W. P., Demaeyer, E. M., and Davies, A. J. S. 1974. Some effects of malnutrition on the immune response in man. *Am. J. Clin. Nutr.* 27:638–646.

Feigenbaum, P. A., Medsger, T. A., et al. 1982. The variability of immunologic laboratory tests. *J. Rheumatol.* 9:408–414.

Fein, B. T., and Kamin, P. B. 1968. Allergy, convulsive disorders and epilepsy. *Ann. Allergy* 26:241–249.

Ferguson, A. C. 1984. Food allergy. Progress in food and nutrition. *Science* 8:77–107.

———. 1978. Prolonged impairment of cellular immunity in children with intrauterine growth retardation. *J. Ped.* 93:52–56.

Forman, R. 1981. Medical resistance to innovation. *Med. Hypotheses* 7:1009–1017.

Foucard, T. 1984. Developmental aspects of food sensitivity in childhood. *Nutr. Rev.* 42:98–104.

Fraker, P. J. 1983. Zinc deficiency: a common immunodeficiency state. *Surv. Imm. Res.* 155–163.

Freedman, B. J. 1977. Asthma induced by sulphur dioxide, benzoate and tartrazine contained in orange drinks. *Clin. Allergy* 7:407–411.

Galland, L. D. 1986. Common-sense models of health and disease. *New Eng. J. Med.* 314:652–658.

Glaser, J., and Johnstone, D. E. 1953. Prophylaxis of allergic disease in the newborn. *JAMA* 153:620–622.

Glatt, M. M. 1986. Alcoholism. *Lancet* 1095–1099.

Golbert, T. M. 1980. Food allergy. *J. Med. Soc. NJ* 77:895–899.

Good, R. A. 1981. Nutrition and immunity. *J. Clin. Immun.* 1:3–11.

———. 1972. Relations between immunity and malignancy. *Proc. Nat. Acad. Sci. USA* 69:1026–1032.

Grandel, K. E., et al. 1985. Association of platelet-activating factor with primary acquired cold urticaria. *New Eng. J. of Med.* 313:405–410.

Gryboski, M. D., and Hillemeier, M. D. 1980. Inflammatory bowel disease in children. *Symposium Inflammatory Bowel Disease* 64:1185–1202.

Halpern, G. W. 1983. Clinical-immunologic correlates: a state of the art review and update. *J. Asthma* 20:251–284.

Hanington, E. 1980. Diet and migraine. *J. of Hum. Nutr.* 34:175–180.

Hay, K. D., and Reade, P. C. 1984. The use of an elimination diet in the treatment of recurrent aphthous ulceration of the oral cavity. *Oral Surg.* 57:504–507.

Hegsted, D. M. 1986. Dietary standards; guidelines for prevention of deficiency or prescription for total health? *J. Nutr.* 116:478–481.

———. 1985. Nutrition: the changing scene. *Nutr. Rev.* 43:357–367.

———. 1982. What is a healthful diet? *Primary Care* 9:445–473.

Hemmings, W. A. 1976. Absorption of dietary protein. *Lancet* 697–704.

———. 1980. First experience of dietary antigen. *Lancet* 818–826.

———. 1978. Food allergy. *Lancet* 608–712.

Hemmings, W. A., and Williams, E. W. 1978. Transport of large breakdown products of dietary protein through the gut wall. *Gut* 19:715–723.

Hilton, P. J. 1986. Cellular sodium transport in essential hypertension. *New Eng. J. Med.* 314:222–229.

Horrobin, D. F., et al. 1979. The nutritional regulation of T lymphocyte function. *Med. Hypothesis* 5:969–985.

Ibero, M., et al. 1982. Dyes, preservatives and salicyclates in the induction of food intolerance and/or hypersensitivity in children. *Allergol. Et Immunopathol.* 10:263–268.

Iyre, R. W., Burton, C. S., and Callaway, J. L. 1984. Urticaria. *NC Med. J.* 45:578–587.

Jackson, P. G., et al. 1981. Intestinal permeability in patients with eczema and food allergy. *Lancet* 1285–1286.

Jacobsen, J. 1984. Learning problems in children—bright kids who fail. *Nursing Times Community Outlook* 219–221.

Jenkins, H. R., et al. 1985. Food allergy the major cause of infantile colitis. *Arch. Dis. in Child.* 59:326–329.

Johnston, P. V. 1985. Dietary fat, eicosanoids, and immunity. *Adv. Lipid Res.* 21:103–140.

Johnstone, D. E., and Dutton, A. M. 1966. Dietary prophylaxis of allergic disease in children. *New Eng. J. Med.* 274:715–719.

Jones, V. A., et al. 1985. Crohn's disease and food sensitivity. *Lancet* 177–180.

Jones, V. A., et al. 1982. Food intolerance: a major factor in the pathogenesis of irritable bowel syndrome. *Lancet* 1115–1117.

Jones, V. A., et al. 1985. Crohn's disease: maintenance of remission by diet. *Lancet* 177–180.

Juhlin, L. 1980. Incidence of intolerance to food additives. *Int. J. Derm.* 19:548–51.

Kailin, E. W., and Hastings, A. 1970. Electromyographic evidence of cerebral malfunction in migraine due to egg allergy. *Med. Ann. Dist. Columbia* 39:437–442.

Kemp, A., and Bryan, L. 1984. Perennial rhinitis—a common childhood complaint. *Med. J. Aust.* 141:640–643.

Kemp, A. S., and Schembri, G. 1985. An elimination diet for chronic urticaria of childhood. *Med. J. Aust.* 143:234–235.

Keusch, G. T. 1984. Indices of immune function in the assessment of human nutriture. *Clin. Nutr.* 3:156–160.

Kirk, R. M. 1986. Could chronic peptic ulcers be localised areas of acid susceptibility generated by autoimmunity? *Lancet* 772–774.

Kjell, A. 1983. The critical approach to food allergy. *Ann. Allergy* 51:256–259.

Knapp, H. R., et al. 1986. In vivo indexes of platelet and vascular function during fish-oil administration in patients with atherosclerosis. *New Eng. J. Med.* 314:937–942.

Kniker, W. T. 1985. The Bela Schick lecture for 1984. Deciding the future for the practice of allergy and immunology. *Ann. Allergy* 55:106–13.

Kutsky, R. J. 1981. *Handbook of vitamins, minerals and hormones.* New York: Van Nostrand Reinhold.

Kushimoto, H., and Aoki, T. 1985. Masked Type I wheat allergy. *Arch. Dermatol.* 121:355–360.

Latham, M. C. 1986. Evolution and infant feeding. *Lancet* 1089–1093.

Law-Chin-Yung, L., and Freed, D. L. J. 1977. Nephrotic syndrome due to milk allergy. *Lancet* 1056–1060.

Lazar, R. H., and Kreindler, J. J. 1985. Allergic causes of pediatric upper airway obstruction. *Ear, Nose and Throat J.* 64:39–46.

Lee, T. H. 1985. The immunopathogenesis and clinical management of food hypersensitivity. *Comp. Ther.* 11:38–45.

Lee, T. H., et al. 1985. Effect of dietary enrichment with eicosapentaenoic

and docosahexaenoc acids on in vitro neutrophil and monocyte leukotriene generation and neutrophil function. *New Eng. J. Med.* 312:1217–
1224.

Lessof, M. H. 1985. Food intolerance. *Proc. Nutr. Soc.* 44:121–125.

————. 1983. Food intolerance and allergy—a review. *Quart. J. Med.* 206:111–
119.

Lessof, M. H., et al. 1980. Food allergy and intolerance in 100 patients—
local and systemic effects. *Quart. J. Med.* 175:259–271.

Levinsky, R. J. 1981. Food antigen handling by the gut. *J. Trop. Ped.* 27:1–
4.

Levinson, A. I. 1984. Urticaria and angioedema. *Postgrad. Med.* 76:183–
192.

Little, C. H., and Stewart, A. G. 1983. Platelet serotonin release in rheumatoid arthritis: a study in food intolerant patients. *Lancet* 297–299.

Locke, S., and Colligan, D. 1986. *The healer within.* New York: E. P. Dutton.

MacLean, L. D. 1979. Host resistance in surgical patients. *J. Trauma* 19:297–
304.

McCarty, E. P., and Frick, O. L. 1983. Food sensitivity: keys to diagnosis.
J. Ped. 102:645–652.

McFarlane, H. 1976. Malnutrition and impaired immune response to infection. *Proc. Nutr. Soc.* 35:263–272.

McFarlane, H., and Hamid, J. 1973. Cell-mediated immune response in
malnutrition. *Clin. Exp. Immunol.* 13:153–164.

McLaughlan, P., and Coombs, R. R. A. 1983. Latent anaphylactic sensitivity
of infants to cow's milk proteins. *Clin. Allergy* 13:1–9.

McMurray, D. N., et al. 1977. Effect of moderate malnutrition on con-
centrations of immunoglobulins and enzymes in tears and saliva of young
Colombian children. *Am. J. Clin. Nutr.* 30:1944–1948.

Malave, I., Nemeth, A., and Blanca, I. 1978. Immune response in malnutrition—effect of protein deficiency on the DNA synthetic response
to alloantigens. *Int. Arch. Allergy Appl. Immun.* 56:128–135.

May, C. D. 1983. Immunologic versus toxic adverse reactions to foodstuffs.
Ann. Allergy 51:267–268.

May, C. D., and Block, S. A. 1978. A modern clinical approach to food
hypersensitivity. *Allergy* 33:166–188.

May, K. L. 1980. Allergy to cereals and dairy products in adult, uncom-
plicated asthma: an epidemiological survey. *Allerg. Immunopath.* 643–
650.

Meeker, H. C., et al. 1985. Antioxidant effects on cell-mediated immunity.
J. Leuk. Biol. 38:451–458.

Meneghini, C. L., and Bonifazi, E. 1985. The role of foods in atopic
dermatitis. *Intl. J. Derm.* 24:158–160.

Mennies, J. H., et al. 1985. An overview of adult allergic disorders. *Nurse Pract.* 16–27.

Metcalfe, D. D. 1984. Diagnostic procedures for immunologically-mediated food sensitivity. *Nutr. Rev.* 42:92–97.

———. 1985. Food allergens. *Clin. Rev. Allergy* 3:331–349.

———. 1984. Food hypersensitivity. *J. Allergy Clin. Immun.* 73:749–762.

Mills, P. R., et al. 1983. Assessment of nutritional status and in vivo immune responses in alcoholic liver disease. *Am. J. Clin. Nutr.* 38:849–859.

Minford, A. M., MacDonald, A., and Littlewood, J. M. 1982. Food intolerance and food allergy in children: a review of 68 cases. *Arch. Dis. Child.* 57:742–747.

Morrow-Brown, H. 1984. A holistic view of allergic disease. *Hum. Nutr.: Appl. Nutr.* 38A:421–434.

Murray, J. J., et al. 1986. Release of prostaglandin D_2 into human airways during acute antigen challenge. *New Eng. J. Med.* 315:800–804.

Neumann, C. G., et al. 1975. Immunologic responses in malnourished children. *Am. J. Clin. Nutr.* 28:89–104.

Nuwayri-Salti, N., and Murad, T. 1985. Immunologic and anti-immunosuppressive effects of vitamin A. *Pharmacol.* 30:181–187.

Ogle, K. A., and Bullock, J. D. 1980. Children with allergic rhinitis and/or bronchial asthma treated with elimination diet: a five-year follow-up. *Ann. Allergy* 44:273–278.

Ogra, P. L., et al. 1984. Interaction of mucosal immune system and infections in infancy: implications in allergy. *Ann. Allergy* 53:523–533.

Palmer, D. L., and Zaman, S. N. 1979. Depression of cell-mediated immunity in cholera. *Infection and Immunity* 23:27–30.

Panush, R. S., and Webster, E. M. 1985. Food allergies and other adverse reactions to foods. *Med. Clin. N. Am.* 69:533–546.

Parke, A. L., and Hughes, G. V. 1981. Rheumatoid arthritis and food: a case study. *Brit. Med. J.* 283:2027–2029.

Pennington, J. A. T., and Church, N. H. 1983. *Bowes and Church's food values of portions commonly used.* 14th ed. Philadelphia: J. B. Lippincott.

Pettigrew, R. A., et al. 1984. Assessment of nutritional depletion and immune competence: a comparison of clinical examination and objective measurements. *J. Parent. Ent. Nutr.* 8:21–24.

Philpott, W. H., and Kalita, D. K. 1980. *Brain allergies.* New Canaan, Conn.: Keats Publishing.

Pietsch, J. B., and Meakins, J. L. 1979. Predicting infection in surgical patients. *Surg. Clin. N. Am.* 59:185–197.

Piness, G., and Miller, H. 1931. The importance of food sensitization in allergic rhinitis. *J. Allergy* 2:73–76.

Podleski, W. K. 1985. Elimination diet therapy in allergic children—a word of caution. *Am. J. Dis. Child.* 139:330–336.

Popescu, I. G. R., Ulmeanu, V., and Murariu, D. 1981. Atopic and non-atopic sensitivity in a large bakery. *Allergol. Immunopathol.* 9:307–312.

Prasad, J. S. 1980. Effect of vitamin E supplementation on leukocyte function. *Am. J. Clin. Nutr.* 33:606–608.

Price, M. L. 1984. The role of diet in the management of atopic eczema. *Hum. Nutr.: Appl. Nutr.* 38A:409–415.

Raffi, M., et al. 1977. Immune responses in malnourished children. *Clin. Immunol. Immunopath.* 8:1–6.

Randolph, T. G., and Moss, R. W. 1980. *An alternative approach to allergies.* New York: Lippincott.

Rapp, D. J. 1979. *Allergies and the hyperactive child.* New York: Simon & Schuster.

Rockwell, S. 1984. *Coping with candida.* Seattle, Wash.: Sally J. Rockwell, Publisher.

Roitt, I. M., et al. 1985. *Immunology.* St. Louis: C. V. Mosby.

Rossiter, M. A. 1985. Food intolerance—a general paediatrician's view. *J. Royal Soc. Med.* Supp. 78:17–20.

Rowe, A. H., and Young, E. J. 1959. Bronchial asthma due to food allergy alone in ninety-five patients. *JAMA* 169:1158–1164.

Rudd, P., Manuel, P., and Walker-Smith, J. 1981. Anaphylactic shock in an infant after feeding with a wheat rusk. A transient phenomenon. *Postgrad. Med. J.* 57:794–795.

Saafinen, V. M., and Kajosaari, M. 1980. Does dietary elimination in infancy prevent or only postpone a food allergy? A study of fish and citrus allergy in 375 children. *Lancet* 166–167.

Saha, K., et al. 1983. Immune deficiency in undernourished children and its correction by nutritional therapy. *Indian J. Med. Res.* 77:73–82.

Sandstead, H. H., et al. 1982. Zinc nutriture in the elderly in relation to taste acuity, immune response, and wound healing. *Am. J. Clin. Nutr.* 36:1046–1059.

Sauberlich, H. E. 1984. Implications of nutritional status on human biochemistry, physiology and health. *Clin. Biochem.* 17:132–142.

Schizgal, H. M. 1981. Nutrition and immune function. *Surg. Ann.* 13:15–29.

Schneider, E. L. 1983. Infectious diseases in the elderly. *Ann. Internal Med.* 98:395–400.

Scrimshaw, N. S. 1977. Effect of infection on nutrient requirements. *Am. J. Clin. Nutr.* 30:1536–1543.

Shambough, Jr., G. E. 1983. Serous otitis: Are tubes the answer? *Am. J. Otol.* 5:63–65.

Sheffy, B. D., and Schultz, R. D. 1979. Influence of vitamin E and selenium on immune response mechanisms. *Fed. Proc.* 38:2139–2143.

Shizgal, H. M. 1981. Nutrition and immune function. *Surg. Ann.* 13:15–29.

Siegel, B. V., and Marton, J. I. 1984. Vitamin C and immunity: influence of ascorbate on prostaglandin E_2 synthesis and implications for natural killer cell activity. *Intl. J. Vit. Nutr.* 54:339–342.

———. 1983. Vitamin C and immunity: natural killer (nk) cell factor. *Intl. J. Vit. Nutr.* 53:179–183.

Smith, M. A., Youngs, G. R., and Finn, R. 1985. Food intolerance, atopy, and irritable bowel syndrome. *Lancet* 1064–1068.

Sprinkle, P. M., McClung, J. E., and Paine, A. J. 1985. The immunocompromised human host: diagnosis and treatment. *Laryngoscope* 95:397–400.

Stiehm, E. R. 1980. Humoral immunity in malnutrition. *Fed. Proc.* 39:3093–3097.

Strauss, R. G. 1978. Iron deficiency, infections and immune function: reassessment. *Am. J. Clin. Nutr.* 31:660–666.

Strober, W., et al. 1976. Secretory component deficiency. *New Eng. J. Med.* 294:351–356.

Swarbrick, E. T., Stokes, C. R., and Soothill, J. F. 1979. Absorption of antigens after oral immunisation and the simultaneous induction of specific systemic intolerance. *Gut* 20:121–125.

Tak, H. L., et al. 1985. Effect of dietary enrichment with eicosapentaenoic and docosahexaenoic acids on in vitro neutrophil and monocyte leukotriene generation and neutrophil function. *New Eng. J. Med.* 312:1217–1224.

Taylor, Jr., W. H. 1980. The do-nothing approach to medical care. *J. Med. Assoc. Alabama* 50:35, 37, 41.

Terr, A. I. 1985. Anaphylaxis. *Clin. Rev. Allergy* 3:3–23.

Thornton, J. R., Emmett, P. M., and Heaton, K. W. 1980. Diet and ulcerative colitis. *Brit. Med. J.* 293–294.

Tolber, S. G. 1981. Food problems. *Cutis* 28:360,2,7.

Van Asperen, P. P., Kemp, A. S., Mellis, C. M. 1984. Relationship of diet in the development of atopy in infancy. *Clin. Allerg.* 14:525–532.

Vinsant, G. O., et al. 1985. Nutritional immunity: a prospective study of thirty-three patients with acute appendicitis. *Am. Surg.* 51:693–696.

Viscomi, G. J. 1975. Allergic secretory otitis media: an approach to management. *Laryngoscope* 85:751–756.

von Krogh, G., and Maibach, H. I. 1981. The contact urticaria syndrome—an updated review. *J. Am. Acad. of Derma.* 5:328–341.

von Schacky, C., Fischer, S., and Weber, P. C. 1985. Long-term effects of dietary marine w-3 fatty acids upon plasma and cellular lipids. Platelet function, and eicosanoid formation in humans. *J. Clin. Invest.* 76:1626–1631.

Wagner, P. A. 1985. Zinc nutriture in the elderly. *Geriatrics* 40:111–125.

Wagner, P. A., et al. 1983. Zinc nutriture and cell-mediated immunity in the aged. *Intl. J. Vit. Nutr.* 53:94–101.

Walker, M. A., and Page, L. 1977. Nutritive content of college meals. *J. Am. Diet. Assoc.* 70:260–266.

Walker, W. A., and Bloch, K. J. 1983. Gastrointestinal transport of the macromolecules in the pathogenesis of food allergy. *Ann. Allergy* 51:240–245.

Walker, W. A., and Isselbacher, K. J. 1974. Uptake and transport of macromolecules by the intestine. Possible role in clinical disorders. *Gastroenterol.* 67:531.

Walker-Smith, J. A., Ford, R. K., and Phillips, A. D. 1984. The spectrum of gastrointestinal allergies to food. *Ann. Allergy* 53:629–636.

Watson, R. R. 1981. Nutrition and immunity. *Assoc. J. Dent. Child.* 48:443–446.

West, R., Maxwell, D. 1984. Food hypersensitivity made life threatening by ingestion of aspirin. *Brit. Med. J.* 228:755–756.

Whitehead, R. 1985. Forms of colitis—a review of recent developments. *Pathol.* 17:204–208.

Wilson, N., and Silverman, M. 1985. Diagnosis of food sensitivity in childhood Asthma. *J. Royal Soc. Med.* Suppl. 78:11–16.

Windham, C. T., et al. 1983. Nutrient density of diets in the USDA Nationwide Food Consumption Survey, 1977–1978: 1. Impact of socioeconomic status on dietary density. *J. Am Diet. Assoc.* 82:28–34.

Windham, C. T., Wyse, B. W., et al. 1983. Nutrient diets in the USDA Nationwide Food Consumption Survey, 1977–1978: II. Adequacy of nutrient density consumption practices. *J. Am. Diet. Assoc.* 82:34–43.

Wing, E. J. 1983. Effect of acute nutritional deprivation on host defenses against listeria monocytogenes—macrophage function. *Adv. Exp. Med. Biol.* 162:245–250.

Woolaway, M. C., Nelson, M., and Herfst, H. 1985. A study of the nutrient content of hospital meals. *Community Med.* 7:193–197.

Workman, E. M., et al. 1984. Crohn's disease and food sensitivity. *Hum. Nutr.: Appl. Nutr.* 38A:469–473.

Worthington, B. S. 1974. Effect of nutritional status on immune phenomena. *JAMA* 65:123–129.

Wright, J. V. 1979. *Dr. Wright's book of nutritional therapy.* Emmaus, Penn. Rodale Press.